Occupational Therapy in Home Health Care

Occupational Therapy in Home Health Care

Catherine Verrier Piersol and Phyllis L. Ehrlich

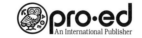
An International Publisher

8700 Shoal Creek Boulevard
Austin, Texas 78757
800/897-3202   Fax: 800/397-7633
www.proedinc.com

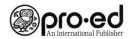

© 2009 by PRO-ED, Inc.
8700 Shoal Creek Boulevard
Austin, Texas 78757-6897
800/897-3202   Fax 800/397-7633
www.proedinc.com

Library of Congress Cataloging-in-Publication Data

Occupational therapy in home health care / [edited by]
Catherine Verrier Piersol and Phyllis L. Ehrlich.
   p. ; cm.
  Includes bibliographical references.
  ISBN-13: 978-1-4164-0403-3
  1. Occupational therapy.   2. Home care services. I. Piersol,
Catherine Verrier, 1959–   II. Ehrlich, Phyllis L., 1952–
  [DNLM: 1. Occupational Therapy. 2. Home Care Services.
3. Patient Care Planning. 4. Practice Management.
WB 555 O1445 2009]
  RM735.4.O23 2009
  362.17'8—dc22
                                    2008030898

Art director: Jason Crosier
Designer: Lissa Hattersley
This book was designed using Adobe Garamond Pro and Neutra

Printed in the United States of America
1   2   3   4   5   6   7   8   9   10   17   16   15   14   13   12   11   10   09   08

Contents

Acknowledgments

From conception to publication, our second edition was a slow but steady work in progress. I am grateful to many individuals who participated in this process. First, I would like to thank PRO-ED, Inc., especially Beth Rowan, for providing ongoing guidance and reassurance as our second edition came together. To my coeditor, Phyllis Ehrlich, and contributing authors, Carol Siebert and Karen Vance, I extend my extreme gratitude for your enthusiasm for this project and the expert knowledge you share in your chapters. As an occupational therapist, I am grateful to the many clients and caregivers with whom I have worked throughout my years of practice. I have learned so much and have so many stories to share. I continue to gain knowledge and glean understanding from my interactions with a diversity of people. I would also like to thank my many colleagues and students for continuously stimulating my desire to learn and expanding my understanding of the therapeutic process. I specifically thank Grace Moses for her contributions to the photos in the patient education materials. Finally, but foremost, I thank my family and friends, who provide the stability in my life, especially my husband, Randy, and my sons, Luke and Joshua, for their never-ending patience and encouragement. Their continuous support constantly reminds me of the importance of home.

Catherine Verrier Piersol

After finishing the first edition, Cathy and I never really thought about doing a second edition to update the material. After we had several conversations in late 2006, we realized that many changes had been made to governmental rules in home care and that uniform terminology was now the practice framework. We could not deny the fact that our book needed a second edition. I would like to thank Cathy for once again including me in this project and for putting forth so much time and effort to coordinate everything. Thanks to Karen and Carol for writing superb chapters and helping us update the information. I would also like to thank my partner, Chris, who has been more than patient and has encouraged me along the way. I must once again thank the patients I have continued to treat over the past several years. They never cease to amaze me in utilizing occupational therapy in home care to help themselves become more independent and functional.

Phyllis L. Ehrlich

Introduction

Occupational Therapy in Home Health Care is a practical resource for occupational therapy practitioners who are interested in or currently work in home health care with adults. The authors have expertise in a range of issues related to home health and provide the practical information occupational therapy professionals need to understand this unique service-delivery area and to establish a successful home care practice. This manual is intended to answer both basic and complex questions, as well as to help the practitioner make informed decisions and choices when faced with challenging practice situations.

Each chapter provides a comprehensive overview of facts and recommendations geared to increasing the practitioner's knowledge. It is not necessary to read the manual cover to cover, as each chapter can stand alone. Cross-references in the text guide readers to related information in other chapters. When applicable, case examples are provided to illustrate specific points.

Chapter 1 explains the nuts and bolts of establishing a home care practice. It answers practical questions such as, What do I need to carry in my car? What credentials do I need? How do I manage my income and expenses? Chapter 2 provides a description of the home care governing systems and the personnel on a home health care team. Understanding the home health industry and its systems is vital for providing effective services, especially given the rapidly changing health care market. Knowing what the important issues are in this field and where to locate more information assists practitioners in staying abreast of the ongoing changes and how various professional groups are responding to them. It is important for professionals to be united and knowledgeable about home care practice to meet the increasing demands.

Chapter 3 provides practical methods for taking an evidence-based approach. Using outcome-based evidence is vital in the effort to promote the profession and to provide skilled services. This chapter provides concrete examples of how an evidence-based approach can be integrated in home health practice. Chapters 4 and 5 delve into the heart and soul of providing services to patients in their homes. The importance of documenting outcomes cannot be overstated. Chapter 4 contains an overview and specific examples of how to clearly and effectively document the intervention being provided, based on the target audience. In home care, the patient's home is the clinic. This raises issues that do not arise in clinic-based practice; it also forces the practitioner to be creative in incorporating different strategies and household objects into the therapeutic process. These issues and more are explored in Chapter 5. (Note that we elected to use the term *patient* to designate the service recipient, the term *caregiver* to denote the family member or other person providing ongoing care and assistance to the patient, and the term *practitioner* to designate the occupational therapist or occupational therapy assistant who provides occupational therapy services.)

This manual would not be complete if it did not address educational opportunities in the area of home health. Chapter 6 provides a format for home health practitioners who wish to establish Level I and/or Level II student programs. Working with patients and caregivers in their familiar environments and enabling them to perform routine tasks offer students a wealth of opportunities to learn the essence of occupational therapy.

The final chapter addresses the issue of planning for discharge, an extremely important component of the home care process. The plan for discharge should be addressed with the patient and caregiver at the initiation of services. The discharge date should never come as a shock to the patient or caregiver.

To assist the patient in following through with therapy goals and the intervention plan, the practitioner typically provides some form of written educational materials. Appendix A shows the 18 reproducible home programs and 3 information sheets, which can be printed and individualized, that are provided on the CD. Appendix B provides a list of resources with Web sites, which is also on the CD. Space is provided for the reader to add new resources as they are discovered.

We hope your experience working in home health is a rewarding one.

Getting Started

Catherine Verrier Piersol, MS, OTR/L

Home health care is an exciting and rewarding area of practice for occupational therapy practitioners. Occupational therapy practitioners are skilled in modifying an individual's environment in order to fit the person's specific needs and abilities. What better environment in which to work than the unique setting of each patient's home? To be successful in home health care, occupational therapy practitioners will find it beneficial to possess strong clinical and time management skills, to understand home health policies, and to enjoy the creativity of occupational therapy practice. This chapter provides the nuts and bolts of getting started. The topics covered in this chapter include the following:

Determining your employment and benefit status

Maintaining your professional credentials and competency

Establishing a contract with an agency

Organizing income and expense records

Purchasing and maintaining your supplies and equipment

Ensuring your safety while on the road

Employment and Benefit Options

When you decide to become a home health care practitioner, you might have a choice of three employment options: regular employee, per diem employee, or independent contractor. Each has advantages and drawbacks, so you must determine which option is best for your circumstances. For example, working as an independent contractor or a per diem employee in home health care while practicing full-time in another arena can be a good way to gain experience and decide whether to commit to full-time home health care practice.

The following overview describes the typical characteristics of the various employment statuses. Because each employer has different policies, it is important to discuss these issues with a prospective employer. If you decide to become an independent contractor, it is also wise to consult your accountant or to request and study the current tax law documents published by the Internal Revenue Service, which has very strict regulations related to employment status.

Regular Employee (Staff)

You are an employee of the agency and receive a pay and benefit package.

The employer expects specific productivity per day and/or week and assigns new cases accordingly. The productivity guideline for full-time status is based on each individual employer and generally ranges between 30 and 40 visits per week.

You are on the employer's payroll and receive a regular paycheck.

You are usually covered by the employer's liability (malpractice) insurance, and workers' compensation and disability income insurance are typically included in your benefit package.

You are usually provided with health insurance benefits and a retirement package.

Per Diem Employee

You are an employee of the agency but typically do not receive a benefits package. You are responsible for managing your own benefits, including insurance and retirement.

Your employer does not require a specific level of productivity, and you have the option to decline referrals offered.

You are on the agency's payroll but are paid only for the visits that you make each pay period (fee-for-service). Employers also frequently reimburse per diem employees for attendance at in-services and staff meetings. Taxes are typically withheld.

You must maintain your own liability insurance (malpractice) and disability income insurance. You are usually covered by workers' compensation.

Independent Contractor (Self-Employed)

You are self-employed and contract your services to an agency for a specific period or project.

You must have contracts with several institutions, companies, or agencies to meet the Internal Revenue Service's conditions on independent contracting.

As your own employer, you determine your own productivity expectation. You may refuse to take a referral.

You are not on the payroll and are paid only for the visits that you make in a given payment cycle (fee-for-service). The payment schedule is outlined in the contract you sign. Your taxes are not withheld.

You receive no benefits and must arrange your own retirement and insurance, including liability insurance and disability income insurance. You are not covered by workers' compensation.

In addition to obtaining health and life insurance, you might want to consider getting disability income coverage. Such insurance provides monthly income if you are unexpectedly unable to work because of a disability, as defined by the policy, for an extended period of time. The cost of disability insurance depends on the policy guidelines (e.g., size of payment per month and length of time you must be disabled before payments begin). The American Occupational Therapy Association provides information on disability income insurance to its members. You also might want to consult your insurance representative.

Questions to Ask as an Employee

Am I responsible for arranging vacation coverage?

How many visits constitute full-time?

Is mileage reimbursed?

Is liability insurance covered?

Are funds available for continuing education?

What is the benefits package?

What is the policy for providing durable medical equipment and assistive devices to patients?

Am I responsible for supervising contract staff, agency employees, or other personnel?

Questions to Ask as a Per Diem Employee

Am I responsible for arranging vacation coverage?

Are equipment and supplies provided?

Am I paid for my time when attending in-services and meetings?

Must I make a minimal number of visits to maintain my per diem status?

Can I refuse a referral?

Is mileage reimbursed?

Am I covered by workers' compensation?

What is the policy for providing durable medical equipment and assistive devices to patients?

Questions to Ask as an Independent Contractor

Am I responsible for arranging vacation coverage?

Am I paid for my time when attending in-services and staff meetings?

Must I take a minimum amount of cases per month?

Preparing for Practice

Table 1.1 provides you with a checklist to guide you in completing the necessary steps involved in establishing a home health practice. If you choose regular or per diem employment, some of these items will not

Table 1.1

Preparing for Home Health Practice

Task	Completed ☑	Date completed
Contact home health agencies to request information regarding potential employment and schedule an interview if indicated. Receive contracts.		
Complete medical clearance (primary care physician).		
Notify auto insurance company of change in vehicle usage.		
Obtain appropriate liability insurance, immunization clearance, and cardiopulmonary resuscitation certification for health professionals.		
Consider disability insurance.		
Complete credential packet to provide to each agency.		
Establish business checking account and gas and credit cards.		
Meet with certified public accountant or tax attorney and set up quarterly tax payments and procedures for maintaining business records.		
Sign contracts (after review by attorney).		
Identify zip codes or counties to which you will travel.		
Set up office space with necessary supplies.		
Design invoice and billing form.		
Purchase supplies and equipment.		
Organize car space with evaluation tools and intervention equipment.		
Obtain office and cell phones.		
Develop plan for familiarizing self with home health care regulations and policies (local, state, and federal).		
Establish resource library and mechanism for searching for evidence to support practice decisions.		
Schedule first patient!		

apply to you. These issues are discussed in further detail throughout the chapter.

Professional Credentials and Competency

As a professional, you are responsible for obtaining and maintaining all the necessary credentials to maintain your license. You must submit the appropriate documentation verifying your credentials to the agencies for which you work, and you must continuously meet all expectations. Although most agencies will notify you when updated documents are due, it is wise to keep your records current. The requirements typically include, but are not limited to, the following:

> Professional license (state regulated)
>
> Certification (National Board for Certification in Occupational Therapy)
>
> Malpractice insurance ($1,000,000 each incident; $3,000,000 aggregate), which is required for per diem employees and independent contractors and recommended for regular employees
>
> Physical or medical clearance and immunizations
>
> Driver's license
>
> Automobile insurance
>
> Cardiopulmonary resuscitation certification for health professionals
>
> Résumé
>
> Evidence of attendance at continuing education sessions and level of competency

The Contract

If you are an independent contractor, you must sign a contract with the agency prior to providing any services. It is standard practice to have an agreement that identifies each party's responsibilities. The contract establishes the foundation on which you do business, so it is important to understand it completely. Having an attorney review the contract is highly recommended. Do not hesitate to seek clarification and modification, if necessary, from the agency representative.

Each contract will have unique language, but the typical components of the contract are as follows:

Responsibilities of the contractor: This section lists responsibilities expected of the occupational therapist, such as maintaining credentials, understanding patient's rights, and knowing the agency's policies and procedures. Specific role restrictions will be listed in this section as well, such as a noncompetition clause, which restricts your right to work for other companies that are in direct competition with your contracting agency.

Responsibilities of the agency: This section lists the duties of the agency, such as offering appropriate referrals, providing consultation and training services, and establishing case management procedures. This section might have a disclaimer stating that the agency makes no representation as to the volume of business to be given to you.

Joint responsibilities: This section describes issues that are mutually binding on both parties, such as an agreement to provide prompt written notice of any changes in the contract and to act in compliance with the various governing bodies.

Payment: This section outlines the terms of payment, such as per-visit reimbursement, fee schedule, and other reimbursed services (e.g., patient conferences and record reviews). You will generally negotiate this visit rate with the agency representative. It is helpful to seek guidance from seasoned practitioners who are willing to share the current rates in your area so you can competitively price your services.

Term of agreement and termination: This section establishes the length of the contract and the procedures for both parties to follow should they wish to terminate it.

Access to books and records: This section specifies the number of years you must retain patient records and make them available to a duly authorized representative of the government. Because of this provision, it is imperative that you properly organize and store your patient records.

Income and Expense Records

Home health care practitioners are responsible for maintaining appropriate records of their work activity. The procedure varies depending on the practitioner's employment status and the institution's policies. Regular employees receive fixed compensation established when the employee is hired. Per diem employees are paid a specific rate per visit, which is established at the date of hire. Thus the amount paid to a per diem employee depends on the number of visits completed in the pay period. Like per diem employees, independent contractors are paid for work completed, but they must invoice the agency to receive payment.

Generally employees (regular and per diem) may utilize the agency's supplies and equipment (e.g., soap, gloves, and evaluation and intervention tools). Self-employed clinicians are responsible for purchasing and maintaining their own supplies and equipment, as well as for paying quarterly estimated federal and state taxes. The cost of most equipment and supplies can be deducted against your taxes as a business expense. Thus if you are self-employed, maintaining accurate income and expense records is imperative.

If you intend to become self-employed, consult with a certified public accountant or tax attorney knowledgeable in self-employment issues. An accountant can guide you in establishing a billing system, understanding the tax laws, and maintaining appropriate records (mileage charts, overhead costs, and income records). Figure 1.1 is an example of an invoice that you can use to bill each agency for services you provide.

Consider establishing a database program that clearly tracks your income and expenses to facilitate the end-of-year tax process. A spreadsheet can be organized vertically by month and horizontally by income or expense item. Typical expenses to track include the following:

Telecommunication: office telephone, cellular telephone, pager

Office expenses: letterhead, envelopes, address labels, business cards, stamps, office supplies

Jane Smith, MS, OTR/L
999-99-9999
1234 E. Oak Street
Springfield, OH 44444
Phone: (555) 555-5252   Fax: (555) 555-5353
E-mail: janes@springoh.net

Invoice for Occupational Therapy Services Home Care

Agency _____ Month _____, 20___

Patient   Dates of Service   Total Visits

Total Visits _____ × _____ = $ _____

Date Submitted _____ Signature _____

Figure 1.1. Independent contractor invoice.

Equipment and supplies: computer and software, printer, fax machine, evaluation tools, intervention equipment

Insurance: disability income coverage, malpractice (liability) insurance, health insurance

Professional expenses: association dues, publication subscriptions, continuing education fees

The most important factor is to establish a system that works for you and maintain it on a daily, weekly, and monthly basis. If you take an organized approach, end-of-year tax preparation will be relatively straightforward.

Supplies and Equipment

Regardless of your employment status, you need to consider the supplies and equipment necessary for managing your practice and providing effective patient care. A well-organized office system and proper record keeping will ensure a foundation for success. As an independent contractor, you might work out of a home-based office and purchase your own supplies. As an agency employee, you might use an on-site office but house some supplies outside the agency walls as well. Table 1.2 lists the standard equipment and business supplies recommended for a successful operation. Typically your car will be your office when you are making visits. Being prepared with the appropriate and required equipment is essential to success. The two right-hand columns in Table 1.2 list items you will want to keep organized in your car and carry into the home when you are on a visit.

Evaluation and intervention are the essences of home health care practice. Before getting started, you should obtain the appropriate evaluation and intervention tools and equipment. As an agency employee, you typically have access to the agency's equipment and must follow the proper procedures for using and maintaining it. As an independent contractor, you are required to purchase your own evaluation and intervention tools.

For the occupational therapist, accurate evaluation procedures and results are crucial for planning intervention. In-home evaluation is typically accomplished through an interview with the patient, family, or

TABLE 1.2
Equipment and Supply Inventory

Office		Vehicle	
Standard equipment	Business supplies	Keep in the vehicle	Take into the home
Computer	Business cards	Street maps	Cell phone
Printer	Invoice	TB mask*	Cardiopulmonary resuscitation mask
Fax machine	Gas card and credit card	Simple tool kit*	
Telephone		Tape measure*	Gloves
File cabinets	Letterhead and envelopes	Instant and/or digital camera*	Blood pressure cuff
	Office supplies		Stethoscope
			Antibacterial soap
			Paper towels
			Antiseptic gel
			Alcohol preps
			Evaluation tools
			Intervention tools

Additional inventory:

Note. The items marked with an asterisk should be taken into the home as needed.

caregivers; your observations; and a formal evaluation. Table 1.3 shows a list of evaluation approaches and intervention strategies, based on the focus of need. It is important to integrate the patient's occupational roles, interests, and habits and the physical, social, and cultural environment into the intervention process. One way to do so is to use everyday activities and items from the patient's home in therapy. Refer to Chapter 5 Table 5.2 for an example of how to assess performance during the initial occupational therapy evaluation visit.

TABLE 1.3
Suggested Evaluation Approaches and Intervention Strategies

Focus of need	Evaluation	Intervention
Performance in areas of occupation (activities of daily living, instrumental activities of daily living)	Occupational performance evaluations Occupational role evaluations Interest evaluations	Assistive devices Equipment catalogs Durable medical equipment
Body functions and performance skills	Goniometer Dynamometer or pinch meter Sensory evaluations Coordination evaluations Cognitive evaluations Performance-based evaluations Perceptual evaluations Stopwatch	Therapy putty Resistive rubber band Pulley Clothespins Nuts and bolts of different sizes Balloons Plastic bowl with rice Soup cans Jars in various sizes Plastic containers with various lids
Contexts	Home safety evaluation Environmental screen	Home modification

You might also consider investing in a supply of assistive devices that patients may try out, and perhaps borrow, to determine whether they will assist with activities of daily living, home management tasks, and leisure activities.

To facilitate the recommendation and provision of durable medical equipment (DME) to your patients, you might find it beneficial to establish relationships with local medical supply companies that are reliable and charge reasonable prices. Also inquire as to whether the company will negotiate a flexible payment plan for patients on fixed incomes. Most companies have catalogs and price lists and might stock certain frequently ordered items. Another useful avenue is to research local organizations that donate equipment to people in need. Examples are equipment-recycling programs operated through rehabilitation hospitals and community organizations that collect, sanitize, and store donated medical equipment, and organizations that assist with the cost of durable medical equipment and/or home modifications.

Equipment Maintenance

Each home health care agency will have operational policies and procedures for sanitation and storage of equipment. The regulations should be documented in a policies and procedures manual. It is your responsibility to familiarize yourself with the agency's policies regarding equipment maintenance and to follow them consistently. This includes cleaning, maintaining, and storing appropriately the supplies and equipment you keep in your vehicle and use for patient care.

Personal Safety Practices

This chapter would not be complete without a discussion of personal safety. As a home health care practitioner, you will work independently and travel alone throughout most of the day. While traveling in the community and entering unfamiliar homes, you will always have the potential to encounter dangerous situations. Safety on the job should always be of utmost importance. Depending on the area of the country in which you live and the type of environment in which you work, personal safety issues may vary. No matter where you are, vigilance and caution are always appropriate.

Make sure to determine where the high-risk areas in your community are and become familiar with the agency's procedures for making visits in those locations. The first principle is to always be prepared and as familiar as possible with the location in which you will be providing services. Will you be working in rural areas where you will be traveling in the middle of nowhere for extended periods of time, or will you be in the heart of a city where you may be walking from door to door? If you will be traveling and working in familiar areas (i.e., near where you live or grew up), step back and try to analyze the area from an outsider's perspective. Identify potentially unsafe areas and situations. If you will be providing services in geographic locations that are unfamiliar to you, take the time to drive through the neighborhoods and note where the police station and firehouse are. Seek specific information from your agency supervisors and refer to and take seriously any materials that are provided as part of the orientation process. Take advantage of any in-service training opportunities offered by the agencies for which you work. Many local police departments offer workshops on personal safety and specific techniques or materials for maintaining safety. Consider the following safety precautions and identify the ones that are appropriate to your situation.

Being Prepared

Be aware of high-risk neighborhoods and seek advice from colleagues and supervisors.

Maintain your automobile to reduce the risk of its developing unexpected mechanical problems.

Always have your cell phone handy.

Keep equipment you will need to take into the home in the front seat rather than in the trunk of your vehicle so you do not have to open the trunk on the street.

Consider carrying a whistle, mace, or another type of deterrent.

Plan your visit schedule ahead of time and be familiar with your travel route between homes.

Phone the patient in advance and ask him or her to be on the lookout for you.

Traveling to the Home

Drive with the doors locked and windows up.

As you approach a home, look for locations where you could seek help if necessary (e.g., business establishment, police or fire station).

Leave nothing visible in your car.

Carry the least possible amount of equipment with you into the home.

Parking Your Car

Avoid traveling down and parking on dead-end streets.

Park your car in a well-lit area near homes or people.

Park your car in an unobstructed area at a distance from any potential hiding places.

Park in the direction you plan on traveling next.

Leaving the Car and Traveling by Foot

Always lock your car.

Carry your keys in your hand when leaving and approaching your car.

If you suspect you are being followed while on foot, call the police.

Do not get out of your car if there is suspicious activity in the area. Leave the area immediately and call the agency and/or the police.

When walking on the street or sidewalk, avoid groups of people.

Walk away from any groups that are blocking entrances or exits.

Approaching the Home

When providing services in apartment buildings, make an effort to introduce yourself to the manager.

Locate the exits in the buildings you enter.

Approach elevators with caution.

Use an empty elevator whenever possible. Stand near the elevator door and the control panel. If you sense danger, push all the floor buttons and exit as soon as possible.

When approaching a house, use the most visible entrance, unless you have been specifically instructed to use a different door.

When first meeting the patient and/or caregiver, introduce yourself and clearly say your name and the name of the agency. If appropriate, show your identification.

Working in the Home Environment

Stay alert at all times when in the home and be aware of other individuals who are in the home.

If you feel threatened by pets in the home, ask the owner to restrain or remove them.

If weapons are visible, request that they be removed from the area during your visit. Notify your supervisor.

Handle yourself with confidence and self-assurance. Do not display fear or insecurity. If you have cause for concern, call the agency once you have left the home and are safely in your car.

Use your common sense and professional judgment while traveling and providing services in the community. Make safety a priority and a habit as you travel from door to door.

Conclusion

This chapter has touched on the important issues you need to consider when getting started in home health care practice and listed the specific items you should have available. The remaining chapters in this manual offer specific information about the knowledge you should possess, the policies and procedures you should understand, and the best practices for performing efficiently and effectively as a home health care practitioner.

The Home Health Industry: Understanding the System

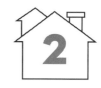

Karen Vance, OTR/L

Health care in the home preceded all other health care settings prior to funding, prior to organized systems, and prior to technology. Though more options for health care delivery are available now than in previous generations, many people prefer to receive health care in the comfort and familiarity of home. Similarly, practicing occupational therapy in the familiar context of the home is inherently more natural for the health care recipient's occupational performance. However, there are many influences on where and how we deliver health care, including policies, regulations, payers, and quality accreditors. There are few better examples than Medicare-certified home health to demonstrate the regulatory impact on occupational therapy practice, as discussed in this chapter. The following sections are designed to provide you with the information necessary to practice optimally in the current setting and to respond to future influences, helping position home health occupational therapy practice for many years to come.

Background

The Health Insurance for the Aged and Disabled Act of 1965 (Title XVIII of the Social Security Act [www.socialsecurity.gov/OP_Home/ssact/title18/1800.htm]), known as Medicare and Medicaid, spearheaded extensive growth in health care over the following 20 years. In response to rates far exceeding average gross domestic product growth, Medicare developed prospective payment systems designed to control health care spending, beginning with hospitals during the 1980s. Diagnosis-

The authors express their gratitude to Missi Zahoransky for her work on this chapter in the previous edition.

related groups shortened hospital stays, as intended, and the percentage of patients discharged to home health services increased significantly. Also during the 1980s, the growth of health maintenance organizations (HMOs) and managed care organizations (MCOs) had an impact on home care services, but Medicare remained the largest single payer for home health. Medicaid and other commercial insurance companies also adhere to many of Medicare's requirements in determining coverage for home health services. Therefore it is extremely important for practitioners to have a clear understanding of Medicare's home care regulations.

Medicare

The Health Insurance for the Aged and Disabled Act, also known as Medicare, was enacted to offer elderly people and people with disabilities health care coverage for hospital, medical, and other health care costs. Supervision of the Medicare program is delegated to the Centers for Medicare and Medicaid Services (CMS), an agency of the U.S. Department of Health and Human Services (HHS). By law, the federal government is not allowed to supervise or control the practice of medicine, so the responsibility for treatment and control of care ultimately rests with the patient, the physician, and the hospital or other facility or agency furnishing the services (CMS, 2003, Pub. 100, Ch. 1, § 20).

The Medicare program provides health care services through two related programs: hospital insurance (Part A) and supplementary medical insurance (Part B). Part A is financed through mandatory payroll contributions by employees and employers. Enrollment in Part B is voluntary and is financed through monthly premiums paid by enrollees and from the general revenue fund of the federal government (CMS, 2003, Pub. 100, § 20.1). Home health is designed to be provided primarily under the Part A benefit.

Medicaid

Medicaid was created to provide health care to people of all ages who meet income limits that qualify them as indigent. Both Medicare and Medicaid were established at the federal level and receive federal funding, but the difference between the two programs is that Medicaid is administered at the state level. The federal government establishes basic guidelines, but each state determines how it will operate its Medicaid program. This means that each state has its own Medicaid criteria and policies, and to participate in Medicaid, a home health agency (HHA) must comply with both the federal guidelines and the regulations of any state in which services are provided.

Occupational therapy practitioners should be aware of the specific guidelines for home care services mandated by the state in which they practice. State Medicaid guidelines are also subject to continual revision, and a strong communication link with the state agency is essential for agencies treating Medicaid patients.

Medicare as Regulator

Medicare stipulates that a home health agency must be a public agency or private organization that is primarily engaged in providing skilled nursing and other therapeutic services. Where applicable, the agency must be approved by the state or local licensing agency as meeting the licensing standards. To participate in the health insurance program, a home health agency must meet certain other requirements included in the law, as well as health and safety conditions prescribed by the secretary of the HHS (CMS, 2003, Pub. 100, Ch. 1, § 10.2).

The Medicare conditions of participation (CoPs) are sets of requirements for acceptable quality in the operation of health care entities. In addition to each condition is a group of related quality standards. The state survey agency ascertains, by a survey conducted by qualified health professionals, whether and how each standard is met. Each provider type is surveyed in accordance with the appropriate protocols based on the substantive requirements in the statute and regulations to determine whether a citation of noncompliance is appropriate. Deficiencies are based on a violation of the statute or regulations, which, in turn, are based on observations of the providers' performance or practices. An institution may fail to comply with one or more of the subsidiary standards during any given survey, but it cannot participate in Medicare unless it meets each and every condition (www.cms.hhs.gov/Survey CertificationEnforcement).

The CoPs implement the requirements of §§ 1861(o) and 1891(a) of the Social Security Act for HHA services and also set forth the additional requirements considered necessary to ensure the health and safety of patients. This means these conditions apply to all patients served by a Medicare-certified home health agency, regardless of who is paying for the services. The following are some of the categories of conditions with which home health agencies must comply:

- personnel qualifications
- patient rights
- confidentiality
- patient liability for payment
- governing body and administration
- personnel policies and contracts
- advisory and evaluation functions, planning, and operating budgets
- physician's plan of care and conformance with physician's orders
- coordination of care
- services provided by individual discipline categories
- initial and comprehensive assessment
- *Outcome and Assessment Information Set* (OASIS) data collection and reporting
- clinical records

The Survey Process

Home health agencies that are certified to participate with Medicare and Medicaid are surveyed on a 12- to 36-month cycle, depending on their previous track record and other defining criteria. In addition, if a complaint is filed against an agency, an emergency survey may be performed. Financial audits and surveys by the fiscal intermediary may be performed at any time throughout the course of participation and can be conducted on-site or through documentation requests.

Compliance surveys consist of on-site visits from state agency representatives (called surveyors), and the survey results are available to the public. The surveyor inspects all aspects of an agency's operations, including policies and procedures, personnel files, patient charts, in-home visits, and any other information the surveyor deems important. Adherence to the CoPs is foremost, as this determines the agency's overall compliance with the regulatory guidelines.

There are two other credentialing bodies in home care: the Joint Commission on Accreditation of Healthcare Organizations (JCAHO) and the Community Health Accreditation Program (CHAP). A home care agency may apply to the CMS for "deemed status," which is approval to participate in the Medicare program based on acceptable ("passing") results of a JCAHO or CHAP survey. The JCAHO and CHAP have their own guidelines and criteria for home care agencies, but CoPs regulations are incorporated into the survey process, and a home health agency must at all times meet the CMS CoPs regulations to be eligible for participation in Medicare or Medicaid.

Medicare as Payer

A person must meet certain criteria to be eligible for coverage of home health services. A person covered by private insurance must meet the criteria of that company, and it is important to determine what these specific criteria are before providing services to such a patient. The Medicare criteria are described here because Medicare is the largest single payer, and many private insurance companies have similar criteria. To qualify for Medicare Part A coverage, a patient must initially meet the following criteria:

- be confined to the home,
- be under the care of a physician,
- be receiving services under a plan of care established and periodically reviewed by a physician, and
- be in need of skilled nursing care on an intermittent basis, physical therapy, or speech-language pathology or have a continuing need for occupational therapy.

For purposes of benefit eligibility, the word *intermittent* makes the distinction between skilled nursing that requires hospitalization versus skilled nursing that can manage the patient's needs at home. The following further explains the coverage criteria:

- The service recipient must be confined to home, a condition referred to as *homebound*. The patient need not be bedridden, but leaving the residence must require a considerable or taxing effort. A residence is wherever the patient makes his or her home and may be the person's own dwelling, a home or apartment, a relative's or caregiver's home, a home for the aged, or another type of institution (e.g., assisted living facility, senior or group home, etc.).

Absences from the home are permitted but must be infrequent in nature, short in duration, or for the purpose of receiving medical treatment. This is an area of dispute for many professionals, because what qualifies as a justified excursion from home is not clearly defined. The regulations state that absences from the home are expected to be related to medical treatment, but other reasons do not negate home care coverage if the excursion is short in duration, is infrequent, and does not indicate that the patient has the capacity to receive health care on an outpatient basis. Documentation must adequately describe the patient's homebound status throughout the certification period so the patient can continue to be eligible for the Medicare home health benefit.

- The patient must be under the regular care of the physician who is qualified to sign the physician certification form and plan of care (CMS, 2003, Pub. 100-2, Ch. 7, § 30.3).
- Services must be provided under a plan of care established and approved by a qualified physician, defined as a doctor of medicine, osteopathy (including osteopathic practitioner), or podiatric medicine who is legally authorized to practice in the relevant state (CMS, 2003, Pub. 100-2, Ch. 7, § 30.2).

The plan of care must contain all pertinent diagnoses, types of services provided including frequency and duration, supplies and equipment needed, mental status, nutritional requirements, medications, safety measures, functional limitations, activities permitted, prognosis, rehabilitation potential, discharge plans, and any other pertinent information the agency deems important to include. For the plan of care, most home health agencies use CMS Form 485 (see Figure 2.1) or a printed version from software that captures all of the required elements.

The physician establishes the plan of care with the assistance of the home health care team. A practitioner of each relevant discipline performs an assessment to determine the best plan of treatment, and with the physician's approval this becomes the patient's plan of care. The orders on a plan of care must reflect the types of service, the professional who

Department of Health and Human Services
Centers for Medicare & Medicaid Services

Form Approved
OMB No. 0938-0357

HOME HEALTH CERTIFICATION AND PLAN OF CARE

1. Patient's HI Claim No.	2. Start of Care Date	3. Certification Period		4. Medical Record No.	5. Provider No.
		From:	To:		

6. Patient's Name and Address

7. Provider's Name, Address, and Telephone Number

8. Date of Birth		9. Sex ☐ M ☐ F	10. Medications: Dose/Frequency/Route (N)ew (C)hanged
11. ICD-9-CM	Principal Diagnosis	Date	
12. ICD-9-CM	Surgical Procedure	Date	
13. ICD-9-CM	Other Pertinent Diagnoses	Date	

14. DME and Supplies	15. Safety Measures:
16. Nutritional Requirements:	17. Allergies

18.A. Functional Limitations	18.B. Activities Permitted		
1 ☐ Amputation	1 ☐ Complete Bed Rest	6 ☐ Partial Weight Bearing	A ☐ Wheelchair
2 ☐ Bowel/Bladder (Incontinence)	2 ☐ Bed Rest BRP	7 ☐ Independent At Home	B ☐ Walker
3 ☐ Contracture	3 ☐ Up as Tolerated	8 ☐ Crutches	C ☐ No Restrictions
4 ☐ Hearing	4 ☐ Transfer Bed/Chair	9 ☐ Cane	D ☐ Other (Specify)
5 ☐ Paralysis 6 ☐ Endurance 7 ☐ Ambulation 8 ☐ Speech 9 ☐ Legally Blind A ☐ Dyspnea With Minimal Exertion B ☐ Other (Specify)	5 ☐ Exercises Prescribed		

19. Mental Status:	1 ☐ Oriented 2 ☐ Comatose	3 ☐ Forgetful 4 ☐ Depressed	5 ☐ Disoriented 6 ☐ Lethargic	7 ☐ Agitated 8 ☐ Other
20. Prognosis:	1 ☐ Poor	2 ☐ Guarded	3 ☐ Fair	4 ☐ Good 5 ☐ Excellent

21. Orders for Discipline and Treatments (Specify Amount/Frequency/Duration)

22. Goals/Rehabilitation Potential/Discharge Plans

23. Nurse's Signature and Date of Verbal SOC Where Applicable:	25. Date HHA Received Signed POT
24. Physician's Name and Address	26. I certify/recertify that this patient is confined to his/her home and needs intermittent skilled nursing care, physical therapy, and/or speech therapy or continues to need occupational therapy. The patient is under my care, and I have authorized the services on this plan of care and will periodically review the plan.
27. Attending Physician's Signature and Date Signed	28. Anyone who misrepresents, falsifies, or conceals essential information required for payment of federal funds may be subject to fine, imprisonment, or civil penalty under applicable federal laws.

Form HCFA-485 (C-3) (02-94) (Printed Aligned)	PROVIDER

Figure 2.1. Home Health Certification and Plan of Care.

will provide each service, and the frequency and duration of
these services (e.g., occupational therapy—two to three times
for 4 weeks [2–3wk4], then one or two times for 3 weeks [1–
2wk3] for activities of daily living [ADL] retraining, instrumental activities of daily living [IADL] retraining, energy
conservation education, functional transfer training, and upper extremity strengthening). A range in the frequency of
visits is acceptable, but be aware that the upper limit of the
range is considered the expected frequency unless the reason
for doing otherwise is well documented. For example, in the
order cited here, three visits are expected each week for the
first 4 weeks of treatment. If the patient receives fewer than
three sessions per week, the provider must document the reason for this (e.g., the patient was ill, the patient was at a doctor's appointment, the frequency was reduced to two times
per week because of patient's progress).

The physician must sign the plan of care, and a home
health agency is not permitted to bill the intermediary for
services until the plan of care has been signed and returned.
Care may be initiated with a verbal order, pending the return
of the signed plan of care. Any change in frequency, treatment regimen, or services provided must be documented
with a written order signed by the physician, which becomes
part of the plan of care. The plan of care must be reviewed
and signed by the physician at least every 60 days (CMS,
2003, Pub. 100-2, Ch. 7, § 30.2).

- The patient must require skilled intermittent nursing care,
  physical therapy, or speech-language pathology services or
  have a continued need for occupational therapy. The patient
  demonstrates a continued need for occupational therapy services when the initial eligibility for home health services has
  been established by virtue of a prior need for skilled nursing,
  physical therapy, or speech-language pathology services in
  the current or prior certification period (CMS, 2003, Pub.
  100-2, Ch. 7, § 30.4). Occupational therapy is recognized as
  a skilled service and may enable the patient to qualify for the
  continuation of home health aide services and medical social
  services.

Consider the following example: A man returns home with a diagnosis of cerebral vascular accident and initially qualifies for nursing, physical therapy, occupational therapy, medical social work, and home health aide services. The patient is discharged from nursing services after 3 weeks, as he is medically stable. The physical therapist discharges him at the end of the first certification period. The occupational therapist documents that continued occupational therapy services are both reasonable and necessary, that the home health aide continues to be necessary for assistance with the patient's care as there are no willing and able caregivers, and that the medical social worker is addressing the patient's future planning needs. By virtue of the occupational therapist remaining on the case (i.e., documenting a continued need for occupational therapy services), the patient would qualify for home care services from the occupational therapist, home health aide, and medical social worker. The HHA must be acting on a physician certification that is part of the plan of care (CMS Form 485) and that certifies the aforementioned criteria for coverage (CMS, 2003, Pub. 100-2, Ch. 7, § 30.4).

Part B outpatient therapy services are a benefit available to home care patients who do not qualify for Part A coverage. To meet Medicare guidelines for outpatient Part B services, the patient must be actively under the care of a physician. Occupational therapy services must follow a plan of care approved, certified, and recertified by the physician. The primary differences between Part A and Part B coverage are that with Part B the plan of care must be reviewed every 30 days and the patient does not need to be homebound.

Reimbursement

Medicare reimburses a home health agency by means of a fiscal intermediary. An intermediary is a public or private agency or organization that has an agreement with CMS to process Part A and Part B Medicare claims for participating providers. In addition to providing reimbursement for services, intermediaries monitor for provision of unnecessary services, furnish consultative services in relation to fiscal data, conduct audits of provider records, assist with the beneficiary appeals process, and serve as a liaison for participating providers (CMS, 2003, Pub. 100, Ch. 1, § 40).

Historically, reimbursement for home health services was covered on a retrospective cost-based method with limits on visit costs. This was essentially a fee-for-service reimbursement system (when a visit was made, it was billed and the agency received compensation). Based on the agency's reported costs, which were reviewed quarterly by the intermediary, a per-visit reimbursement charge was established up to a "reasonable and necessary" cap. At the end of the fiscal year, the agency completed an annual cost report, and any miscalculations were adjusted. The agency was reimbursed only the cost of doing business; it was not meant to make a profit.

Currently, home health is paid under a prospective payment system (PPS). This system shifted the payment for services from retrospective cost-based *reimbursement* to prospective *payment*. A dollar amount is paid to the agency for a 60-day episode of care. The dollar amount is based on the regional wage index for the area where the beneficiary lives and is individualized to the patient by data collected during the comprehensive assessment. These data predict the amount of resources necessary to provide adequate service to the patient for the 60-day episode. If the agency uses more resources than predicted for this period of time, there is a margin of loss for that episode. If the agency reaches the goals stated on the plan of care, using less than the dollar amount provided, then the agency's margin is a profit for that episode.

Payments are split so agencies receive 60% of the projected payment at the beginning of the first episode (50% for the beginning of subsequent episodes) and the remaining balance when the final claim is filed. The final payment reflects changes based on the following adjustments: low utilization payment adjustment (LUPA), which occurs when fewer than five total visits are made by the agency; significant change in condition (SCIC), which occurs when the patient has an unanticipated change not foreseen at the plan of care; partial episode payments (PEP), which occur when the patient elects to transfer to another agency or is discharged with all goals met but returns to any home health agency before the 60-day episode ends; and outliers, which occur when an adjustment is made when the costs for the episode exceed the projected payment by a certain percentage—however, this adjustment is intended to cover only a portion of the additional cost.

Medicaid and Commercial Insurance Reimbursement

Medicaid reimbursement procedures vary from state to state. Each agency must work with state agencies and provide specific financial documents to establish the billing rates for home care services. The greatest variability lies in private insurance coverage, because each agency develops contractual arrangements specifying predetermined rates for each service provided. It is very important to be aware of the surrounding market when pricing services, because bidding too high can bar an agency from coverage under a particular insurance company, MCO, or HMO, whereas pricing services too low can make an HHA's margin of loss too great. Many commercial insurance companies require preauthorization for home care services, and visits are frequently authorized in small increments, with frequent written or verbal updates required to continue coverage.

Consider this example: A patient with private insurance is discharged from the hospital and needs occupational therapy. The provider submits a preauthorization request for the service. The insurance company approves one occupational therapy evaluation and requests an update on the patient's needs prior to authorizing treatment. The therapist performs the evaluation and completes the required update. The insurance company approves three visits, after which a second update is required to continue treatment. Visits may continue to be authorized in such small increments until the therapist discharges the patient or the insurance company denies future treatment.

Principles Governing Reasonable and Necessary Occupational Therapy Services

The *Medicare Benefit Policy Manual* (CMS, 2003, Pub. 100) delineates five basic principles that govern eligibility for occupational therapy services. These principles are frequently used by other payer sources as well for guidelines to determine authorization:

1. The patient requires skilled occupational therapy if the complexity of the service can be performed safely and/or effectively only by or under the supervision of a skilled therapist.
2. The assessment, development, and implementation of a patient's plan of care require skilled therapy intervention. The plan is signed by a physician, and it meets the patient's needs.
3. The skills of a therapist are valid to treat the illness or injury. The medical condition is an important factor but should never be the sole factor in deciding whether skilled therapy is necessary. This is frequently an important factor in occupational therapy because the patient may be treated for a condition that results from a preexisting illness.
4. A nonskilled service may become skilled in nature if, because of special medical considerations or complications, treatment by skilled personnel becomes necessary.
5. The skilled therapy must be reasonable and necessary for the treatment of the patient's illness or injury. This means that the type of treatment and its frequency must be consistent with the severity and nature of the patient's diagnosis. The service provider must also document that the patient's condition can be expected to improve in a reasonable and generally predictable period of time or that the skilled service is necessary to establish, implement, and monitor a safe and effective maintenance program (CMS, 2003, Pub. 100-2, Ch. 7, § 40.2.1).

Denials and Appeals

Fiscal intermediaries randomly audit bills for compliance and accuracy. A person knowledgeable in billing procedures is a critical staff member, as the financial solvency of the agency may depend on him or her. It is important to be aware of a few basic facts about denials:

- Every reimbursement source must have an appeals policy in place.

- Many denials are overturned in favor of the health care professional when an appeal is submitted in a timely manner and supported by complete documentation.
- Many occupational therapists are not informed of denials. Familiarize yourself with the reimbursement process in your facility, agency, or practice and ensure you have access to any denials involving occupational therapy.

Keep the following in mind when submitting a claim to help avoid a denial:

- Review all documentation before submitting it. Many denials are based on poor or insufficient documentation of the treatment.
- Ensure that all notes are properly signed and cosigned. Entire claims have been denied for failing to meet this requirement.

If a claim is denied, take the following steps:

- Find out the appeal process for the reimbursement source that denied your claim.
- Ascertain the specific reasons for the denial. Many denials result from practitioners' making errors during the billing process, missing deadlines, or following incorrect procedures.
- Review the appeal in a timely manner.
- If you lose an appeal, try to find out the specific reason why, to avoid future denials.
- Be prepared. An appeal takes time and effort.
- Involve yourself in all occupational therapy denials and provide necessary documentation for a successful appeal.

Influences on Home Health Occupational Therapy Practice

Policy initiatives, payment methodologies, the health care market, and technology are among the many influences on when, where, and how occupational therapists practice. For example, the policies that created federal funding for health care in 1965 greatly increased occupational therapy in many health care settings. However, the payment methodology of cost-based reimbursement in home health greatly influenced the underutilization of occupational therapy in this particular health care setting for many years. As described earlier, the cost-based reimbursement system was an incentive for home health agencies to make as many visits as possible to keep agency costs under the limit. This affected practice patterns by encouraging practitioners to increase the number of home health aide visits and keep patients on service as long as the patient met the coverage criteria. A patient achieving independence in ADL would not meet the need for continuing personal care provided by a home health aide. Therefore occupational therapy practitioners lost opportunities to help assist patients to remain in their own homes with less or no assistance.

However, other changes have since begun to influence health care delivery, such as outcomes quality research during the 1980s; the Balanced Budget Act of 1997 and PPSs in long-term care, home health, and hospital outpatient facilities bringing new financial incentives; evidence-based practice research; and technology for improved data management and health care delivery. Home health operations and practices that have already been, and will be, changed by these influences are discussed in the following sections.

Outcome-Focused Health Care

Medicare commissioned the University of Colorado Health Sciences Center's Center for Health Services Research (CHSR) to develop a system of measuring home health quality by the outcomes achieved. By 1999, the first piece of the quality improvement process was ready and mandated for all Medicare-certified home health agencies. This was the measurement piece of outcomes monitoring, called the *Outcome and Assessment Information Set* (OASIS) (www.cms.hhs.gov/OASIS/).

The updated comprehensive assessment and OASIS regulations appear in the January 25, 1999, *Federal Register* (CMS, 1999) as a CoP for home health agencies. The standards stipulate that all patients must receive a specific, comprehensive assessment that accurately reflects the patient's current health status and includes information that may be used to demonstrate the patient's progress toward achievement of desired outcomes. The comprehensive assessment must identify the patient's continuing need for home care and meet the patient's medical, nursing, rehabilitative, social, and discharge planning needs and must be completed within the first 5 days of the start of care. For Medicare beneficiaries, the HHA must verify the patient's eligibility for the Medicare home health benefit, including homebound status.

The standard continues that a registered nurse must complete the comprehensive assessment when nursing is on the orders. When physical therapy, speech-language pathology, or occupational therapy is the only service ordered by the physician, practitioners of any of these disciplines may complete the comprehensive assessment. The occupational therapist may complete the comprehensive assessment if the need for occupational therapy establishes program eligibility. Because occupational therapy is not a qualifying discipline for the Medicare Part A home health benefit, it does not establish program eligibility for a Medicare PPS patient. If occupational therapy establishes eligibility for other insurances, then an occupational therapist may complete the comprehensive assessment for that patient if nursing is not on the initial orders.

As CoPs, OASIS data were initially mandated to be collected on all adult nonmaternity patients regardless of the payer source. Later, there was a temporary hold on the requirement to collect or transmit data on non–Medicare/Medicaid patients. These data are submitted electronically to state agencies and required by regulation to be integrated into comprehensive assessments completed at the following time points:

- start of care
- resumption of care following an inpatient stay
- recertification (follow-up) assessment during the last 5 days of the episode
- other follow-up for a significant change in patient's condition
- transfer to an inpatient facility
- discharge from an agency or death at home

Refer to Chapter 3 for an additional discussion of OASIS data collection or consult the OASIS page on the CMS Web site at www.cms.hhs.gov/OASIS.

OASIS and PPS

Medicare was designing prospective payment for home health as the research was simultaneously being done for the outcome measurement system. Some of the OASIS items had predictive value for the amount of resources a HHA would need to provide care to that patient for that 60-day episode. OASIS data collection was then mandated as home health shifted into PPS, becoming part of the payment system. Twenty-three of the OASIS items became the case-mix data elements that individualized the payment to that patient. These case-mix data are categorized into three domains: clinical, functional, and service utilization. The three domain scores determine to which of the 80 home health resource groups (HHRG) the patient will be assigned for payment. One of the clinical domain items is the patient's primary home care diagnosis, including the corresponding code from the ICD-9 coding manual. The *International Classification of Diseases, 9th Revision, Clinical Modification* (ICD-9-CM) is used to code and classify morbidity data from health care settings. For this reason, understanding the coding process has become a critical skill set for all practitioners in home health.

The CHSR reported high interrater reliability results for OASIS data collection during its research, yet OASIS training among HHAs varies greatly, so it is imperative that agencies strive to increase consistency among all who collect the data. Occupational therapists must take an active role in understanding accurate data collection and how to contribute even when not completing the assessment. Inaccurate data collection can lead to inaccurate episode payments and, more important, inaccurate outcomes.

Home Health Quality Initiative

The OASIS collects measurement outcomes, which quantifies the change in the patient's health status between two or more time points. These outcome measures are the basis for outcome-based quality improvement (OBQI), which is a systematic approach HHAs can implement to continuously improve the quality of care they provide. Agencies receive reports from the Web site through which OASIS data are transmitted. The reports give agencies risk-adjusted statistics on their outcomes compared to their own data from a prior time frame and to national averages. Comparisons are identified when the outcomes that are above or below averages are statistically significant. OBQI is designed to use the information on these reports to identify which outcome measures, such as improvement in bathing, the agency should target for improvement. Once an outcome measure is targeted, the care producing the outcome is investigated; best practices are researched, developed, and implemented; and results are monitored. Most agencies develop OBQI committees to review, identify, investigate, and plan for quality care. These committees then provide results and recommendations to the rest of the agency. Occupational therapy practitioners can provide valuable insight as a committee member and should participate in this process. The OBQI model was originally presented as a circle, emphasizing the continuous quality improvement cycle.

Home Health Compare

Since fall 2003, the CMS has posted on www.medicare.gov a subset of OASIS-based quality performance information showing how well home health agencies assist their patients in regaining or maintaining their ability to function. Measures of how well people can get along in their homes performing ADL form a core of the measures, but these are supplemented with questions about physical status and two use-of-service measures (hospitalization and emergent care) (www.cms.hhs.gov/HomeHealthQualityInits/). Consumers are able to choose one agency and see how the quality indicators compare to state and national averages, or they can compare multiple agencies within a selected area.

Future CMS Priorities

The CMS posts several new priorities that are expected to influence planning for the future:

- utilize **pay for performance,** which ties a portion of reimbursement to delivery of care that has proved to be effective;
- **standardize assessment and quality measurement** across (postacute) health care settings;
- **integrate measures of process and systems;** and
- use **electronic health records.**

Pay for performance logically will link to actual activities and efforts of providers—using evidence-based practices and systems (in the

form of structural measures that will be collected at the agency level)—
to promote use of such practices. Planning and discussions are in a pre-
liminary phase. Providers, consumers, and interested parties, such as the
many organizations that represent and work with patients in post-acute,
home, community, and long-term care settings, will be part of these efforts as they evolve (www.cms.hhs.gov/HomeHealthQualityInits/).

Quality Improvement Organizations

Part of the quality initiative includes quality improvement organizations
(QIOs). QIOs exist in each state and are private organizations that contract with the CMS to help improve the quality of care provided to
Medicare patients. In addition to assisting beneficiaries with complaints
about the quality of care they receive, physicians and other health care
experts work with home health agencies to encourage the adoption, use,
and monitoring of best practices and quality measures. QIOs in each
state promote awareness, understanding, and use of this information by
working with intermediaries, including discharge planners, community
organizations, and the media. QIOs began phasing in assistance to home
health agencies seeking to improve performance on quality measures in
August 2002 (www.cms.hhs.gov/HomeHealthQualityInits/).

The QIO program takes its lead from the Institute of Medicine
(IOM) by defining best practice as *the right care for every person every
time.* The CMS program assists providers in transforming quality to
make health care safe, effective, patient centered, timely, efficient, and
equitable. The overall program vision is designed to transform health
care quality using the following strategies (www.cms.hhs.gov/Quality
ImprovementOrgs/):

- measure and report performance,
- adopt health care information technology and use it
  effectively,
- redesign the process, and
- transform the organizational culture.

These CMS initiatives influenced a significant change in home health
payment methodologies and approach to quality care management in

the beginning of the 21st century and promise to continue its effect on health care in general going forward.

The Home Care Team and Coordination of Services

The PPS method of payment for home care services has greatly influenced the need for the coordination of services to ensure efficient and cost-effective treatment. To provide cost-effective care, a home care team must accurately assess all patients and determine the best skill mix of disciplines to assist the patient in managing his or her own health needs. It is now incumbent on the agency to assess that all service utilization within the 60-day episode is weighed against the value it brings to the patient's outcome. The collaborative team approach to care allows agencies to cost efficiently achieve good outcomes. The CMS included patient-centered care in the vision of transforming health care. Including the patient in the home health team will then be a critical component of achieving *sustainable* outcomes to assist the patient in managing his or her own health needs.

Although each member writes different goals specific to his or her profession and areas of expertise, the home care team shares the same fundamental goal of helping the patient function safely and remain in the home setting. When all team members understand each other's roles, the most effective skill mix can be applied and, even more important, integrated. Each discipline must understand its own value and communicate it well to each other and the agency.

The key to any effective team effort is communication. Good communication facilitates cohesiveness in the patient's treatment and, most important, increases the chance of successful patient and agency outcomes. Technology continues to influence and add vehicles for team communication. Weekly staff meetings to discuss patients are very helpful, but other commonly used modes of communication are pagers, cell phones, voice mail, e-mail, faxes, and written communication forms. Each agency and its personnel will develop their own system for communication, but some means of team collaboration are fundamental to managing good care.

The Team Players

Typical members of a patient's health care team include the following:

patient
physician
case manager
nurse (including specialties
    such as IV, behavioral health,
    maternal health)
occupational therapist and
    occupational therapy
    assistant
dietician
durable medical equipment
    and medical supply
    representative

family and caregivers
intake coordinator and staff
clinical supervisor or manager
physical therapist and
    physical therapy assistant
speech-language pathologist
home health aide
medical social worker
pharmacologist
office support staff
financial advisor or manager
ethics committee

Many referrals for home care will be initiated without the inclusion of occupational therapy. It is imperative that occupational therapy practitioners be willing and able to market their services, document cost-effectiveness and efficacy, and, most important, be a valuable team member. The process of education and team building occurs over time and is a continual work in progress. Occupational therapy practitioners who demonstrate a high degree of professionalism in dealings with other team members ultimately will receive increased referrals.

Occupational therapy practitioners must also be willing to serve as volunteers on agency committees and action groups. Most agency decisions are made internally by a small group of people yet affect the entire team. Home care administrators are open to input from the entire team but may not proactively recruit individual members, and occupational therapists need to take the initiative to step forward. A good example is the OBQI committee, as discussed earlier.

Some agencies and many software vendors are designing care paths. When possible, input from the occupational therapist is vital in this process as well. These care paths may be called by many names (e.g., clinical pathways, team plans, diagnostic treatment plans, protocols, etc.), but they all serve the same purpose: to anticipate a patient's course of treatment prior to admission to the home care agency. Without appropriate input, occupational therapy may be overlooked as a viable part of a care path.

The emphasis on outcomes creates an enormous opportunity to advance the provision of occupational therapy services in home care. By educating other professionals about the unique and important services they offer, occupational therapists can become vital team members involved in many aspects of the home care agency.

Maintaining Professional Relationships and Networking

It is vital to the very existence of occupational therapy that practitioners continuously network, develop, and maintain professional relationships. Changes are inevitable in the health care market, and as professionals we have a responsibility to be prepared for these changes. Being informed and knowledgeable is crucial to the continued growth of our profession. Some of the most common means of networking are to participate in the following:

- professional consortia
- national, state, and local occupational therapy associations
- national and state health care associations
- agency committees
- Internet communications (e-mail, Listservs, chat rooms, etc.)

Conclusion

Occupational therapy practitioners who practice in the home understand the opportunities for improving occupational performance within the rich context of the patient's natural environment. The pragmatic context of the environment, however, can influence whether the practitioner is able to apply his or her clinical reasoning expertise in the manner he or she chooses. Therefore an understanding of that environment and the system and its players is paramount for the occupational therapy practitioner to optimize his or her own effectiveness, with individual patients and with HHAs and the larger community. Advocating for optimized occupational therapy opportunities improves the health of patients and the profession.

A Practical Approach to Evidence-Based Practice

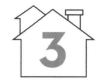

Catherine Verrier Piersol, MS, OTR/L

Evidence-based medicine, as originally defined by its founders, is "the conscientious, explicit and judicious use of current best evidence in making decisions about the care of individual patients" (Sackett, Richardson, Rosenberg, & Haynes, 1997, p. 2). Subsequently, the authors modified their definition of evidence-based medicine to encompass "the integration of best research evidence with clinical expertise and patient values" (Sackett, Strauss, Richardson, Rosenberg, & Haynes, 2000, p. 1). This revised definition acknowledges the expertise the practitioner brings to the practice encounter and the individual values, interests, and goals of the patient. In occupational therapy, evidence-based practice (EBP) can be defined as the process of assessing and utilizing current research information to design and implement intervention that is effective and efficient and has a positive impact on the patient's quality of life and his or her ability to participate in day-to-day occupations. In other words, as an occupational therapist you strive to provide the best type of treatment using the most current knowledge. When working with a patient, do you ask yourself, "What would be the best treatment or intervention for my patient?" or "I wonder if there is a better type of intervention that would be more effective with my patient?" Seeking answers to questions like these is an example of an EBP approach. Occupational therapists must determine the most appropriate and effective evaluation or intervention method, technique, or protocol based on the best current evidence (research). It is essential that you, as an occupational therapy practitioner, integrate EBP methods into your practice toolbox to ensure the viability of the profession (Tickle-Degnen, 2000b).

Portions of this chapter are from "Integrating Evidence-Based Practice in Home Health," by C. V. Piersol, 2005, *Home and Community Health Special Interest Section Quarterly, 12,* pp. 2–4. Copyright 2005 by the American Occupational Therapy Association, Inc. Reprinted with permission.

Regardless of the service delivery setting, we must make using evidence to support clinical reasoning and practice decisions second nature if we are to be accountable for our services and meet the challenges of practice in the 21st century (Stube & Jedlicka, 2007; Tickle-Degnen, 1999). EBP encompasses a set of methods that must become part of our everyday approach to treating a patient in the home. You may be thinking, "Of course I should be using the best type of intervention or the treatment method that has been shown to be effective through research, but how do I stay on top of all that information?" The American Occupational Therapy Association (AOTA) responded to this call with the Evidence-Based Literature Review Project (Lieberman & Scheer, 2002). The project seeks "to develop a series of evidence-based literature reviews of occupational therapy's effectiveness with health conditions addressed in AOTA's Practice Guidelines" (Lieberman & Scheer, 2002, p. 344). The AOTA Evidence-Based Practice Resource Directory is available online (www.aota.org/Educate/Research.aspx). As a member of AOTA, you are able to use this resource directory to locate evidence that will assist in your treatment planning process and also provide you with information to share with patients, caregivers, and physicians.

So how do you fit this approach into your practice routine? How do you integrate EBP into your typical day on the job? The occupational therapy literature describes the EBP process, emphasizing the importance and necessity of using evidence in practice, and presents a framework for advancing the integration of EBP into our daily habits as occupational therapists (Abreu, 2002; Holm, 2000; Kielhofner, 2005; Law, 2000; Law & MacDermid, 2008; Tickle-Degnen, 1999, 2000a, 2000d).

The remainder of this chapter provides practical methods for using an EBP approach in home health practice.

Implementing an Evidence-Based Practice Approach

To provide an objective and systematic approach for integrating evidence into daily practice decisions, occupational therapists should use an organized approach (Rosenberg & Donald, 1995; Sackett et al., 1997; Tickle-Degnen, 2000b). The five-step approach listed below is easily applied to the occupational therapy process:

1. identify a practice or clinical question,
2. gather current research evidence,
3. analyze and critique the evidence,
4. integrate the evidence into practice, and
5. evaluate the effectiveness of the evidence-based practice.

The following is a description of each of the five steps as they apply to occupational therapy, followed by a case example.

1. *Identify a practice or clinical question—the question relates to the patient situation.* Identify a question that relates specifically to the patient you are treating. Using client-centered principles (Law, Polatajko, Baptiste, & Townsend, 1997) reflect on the patient's occupational performance abilities and limitations, unique sociocultural contexts, and self-identified goals. When forming the practice question, consider intervention that will *encourage participation in activities that have the most meaning for the patient.* It may be helpful to use the PICO method when identifying the key components of the question (Richardson, Wilson, Nishikawa, & Hayward, 1995). The PICO method is as follows:

P = *Person:* Identify the patient (condition, problem).

I = *Intervention:* Describe the intervention that is under investigation.

C = *Comparison:* Describe a comparative intervention. (There might not be one, so this element might not be included in the question.)

O = *Outcome:* Describe the outcome of choice.

Once you form the question, your next step is to search for evidence.

2. *Gather current research evidence to answer the question.* You can find evidence in many ways. Doing an online literature search is one method. This approach requires a working knowledge of search engines, key words, and methods for targeting the search. As a home care therapist, you might have demands that can limit your ability to perform an extensive literature search. In response to occupational therapists' growing need to base practice decisions on empirical evidence, and given the time demands of their daily practice, the

AOTA launched the Evidence-Based Literature Review Project to provide easy-to-read summaries of articles selected from the scientific literature (Lieberman & Scheer, 2002). This project has resulted in the *Evidence-Based Practice Resource Directory* (AOTA, 2008). The resource directory is an online service (www.aota.org/Educate/Research/EvidenceDirectory.aspx) that links users to Internet sites related to the EBP of occupational therapy. The resource directory is organized to connect occupational therapists, occupational therapy assistants, and students with useful Web-based resources, including

- databases and Internet sites in occupational therapy, rehabilitation, and health outcomes;
- tutorials for acquiring basic- and intermediate-level skills to search and interpret the literature relevant to occupational therapy; and
- national and international evidence-oriented Internet sites posted by universities, government agencies, and private organizations.

Similar to the AOTA's resource is the Cochrane Library of reviews, which is an excellent resource for evidence (www.cochrane.org). The Cochrane Library is continually updating its evidence and has increasingly more occupational therapy–based reviews. Both the AOTA directory and the Cochrane Library provide a summary of the article, its relevance, and its indications for practice. Starting with these resources for evidence is an efficient approach to seeking evidence to answer your clinical questions.

In addition, you can perform a literature search using the following databases:

- OT Search: www.aota.org/otsearch (subscription only)
- OTseeker: www.otseeker.com
- Current Index to Nursing and Allied Health Literature (CINAHL): www.cinahl.com
- PubMed: www.ncbi.nlm.nih.gov/sites/entrez/
- LexisNexis: http://web.lexis-nexis.com
- ProQuest: http://proquest.com

Tickle-Degnen (2000b) effectively described other methods for gathering evidence. In her EBP forum, Tickle-Degnen (2000b) suggested other activities that constitute evidence-based practice approaches:

- Attend continuing education workshops. Keep a record of your continuing education. Maintain a database of evaluation tools and intervention methods that relate to your practice areas.
- Join professional Listservs. The Home and Community Health Special Interest Section Listserv is an example (www.aota.org/Practitioners/GetInvolved/Listservs.aspx).
- Join a journal club in which you read and discuss current literature.
- Maintain a database of current literature organized by practice question, key word, or topic area.

Once you uncover the evidence through these various methods, your next step involves evaluating the quality of the evidence.

3. *Analyze and critique the evidence-based evaluation and/or intervention.* The validity, reliability, and usefulness of the evidence must be evaluated. The analysis process is used to establish the quality of the evidence and to determine which evidence best answers the practice question. The following online resources provide guidelines for this process:

- AOTA Evidence-Based Practice Resource Directory: www.aota.org/Educate/Research/Evidence.aspx
- Evidence-Based Medicine Tool Kit: www.med.ualbrta.ca/
- The Cochrane Collaboration Training Resources: www.cochrane.org/resources/training.htm
- Evidence-Based Practice Forum: "What Is the Best Evidence to Use in Practice?" (Tickle-Degnen, 2000b)

Through the analysis process you should also be gaining knowledge to use to explain the evidence to the patient, caregiver, physician, other team members, and third-party payer. You must be able to explain the evidence in both professional terminology and layman's terms.

The next step is to use the evidence!

4. *Integrate the evidence into the evaluation and/or intervention plan.* Once you locate and critique the evidence, you must then implement and utilize it to guide your practice decisions. Again, part of this process is being able to explain what you are doing with your patient and the caregiver.

5. *Evaluate the effectiveness of the evidence-based evaluation and/or intervention.* It is vital that you assess the effectiveness of the intervention and provide proper documentation (Tickle-Degnen, 2000c). Chapter 4 provides specific guidelines for effective documentation in home health practice.

Case Story: Mrs. Richards

The following case story provides a concrete example of the methods for and outcomes of using an EBP approach in home health.

Mrs. Richards was diagnosed with a left cerebral vascular accident (CVA) after experiencing weakness on her right side. Once medically stable, she was admitted to an inpatient rehabilitation unit and received occupational therapy, physical therapy, and speech therapy. She was discharged home with a referral for home health occupational therapy. The occupational therapist has received many similar referrals. She questions the approach she will take to treat this individual after she completes the evaluation and develops the problem list; the patient and family express their goals. The following table provides an example of how the occupational therapist integrates the use of evidence into her daily practice using the five steps.

Evidence-based practice step	Case example: Mrs. Richards
1. Identify a practice or clinical question—the question relates to the patient situation.	PICO method: **P** = *Person:* an individual with CVA **I** = *Intervention:* use a functional or compensatory approach during treatment **C** = *Comparison:* use a sensorimotor approach during treatment **O** = *Outcome:* maximize the level of independence in person's ability to dress Question: For Mrs. Richards, who is post-CVA (>1 month) and being treated in her home, will using a functional or compensatory approach instead of a sensorimotor approach increase her independence in dressing?

Evidence-based practice step	Case example: Mrs. Richards
2. Gather current research evidence to answer the question.	The occupational therapist starts by looking at the AOTA Evidence-Based Practice Resource Directory for literature related to the question: • Functional treatment may be as beneficial as sensori-motor integration (Jongbloed, Stacey, & Brighton, 1989). • Practice in dressing may improve stroke patients' dressing skills (M. F. Walker, Drummond, & Lincoln, 1996). • Purpose may enhance stroke patients' upper-limb performance (Nelson et al., 1996). In addition, a search on PubMed gleans the following information: • The influence of cognition on a person's ability to learn compensatory strategies has implications for the design of rehabilitation therapies (C. M. Walker, Sunderland, Sharma, & Walker, 2004). • Adding a specific intervention for the arm during the acute phase after a stroke resulted in a clinically meaningful and long-lasting effect on motor function. The effect can be attributed to early, repetitive, and targeted stimulation (Feys et al., 2004).
3. Analyze and critique the evidence-based evaluation and/or intervention.	On the basis of the literature, the occupational therapist uses the guidelines presented in the "AOTA Continuing Education Article" (Holm, 2001) and information presented in the AOTA Evidence-Based Practice Resource Directory to decide to take more of a compensatory approach, taking into consideration the cognitive ability of Mrs. Richards and incorporating daily practice into her routine. A summary of the evidence and the reasons for certain intervention activities and approaches are explained to Mrs. Richards and her family, who are in agreement.
4. Integrate the evidence into the evaluation and/or intervention plan.	The occupational therapist and Mrs. Richards work together to determine the specific compensatory strategies that best help Mrs. Richards gain independence in dressing. By accurately and concisely documenting Mrs. Richards's progress and using the evidence gathered during the literature review, the occupational therapist is able to justify 14 total occupational therapy visits. *(continues)*

Evidence-based practice step	Case example: Mrs. Richards
5. Evaluate the effectiveness of the evidence-based evaluation and/or intervention.	Outcome-based documentation is imperative to justify and provide evidence of the benefits of occupational therapy. The occupational therapist's documentation included initial evaluation results with specific client-centered targeted goals and clinical notes that provided objective data indicating improved patient performance based on the established goals. Mrs. Richards was able to learn one-handed dressing techniques and use a button hook to become independent in dressing.

Outcome-Based Quality Improvement as Evidence

In addition to using the process described here, occupational therapists and occupational therapy assistants can use their home care agency's outcome-based quality improvement (OBQI) reports as evidence that their occupational therapy interventions are effective (Centers for Medicare and Medicaid Services, 2002). Through a retrospective analysis of the agency's OBQI reports, practitioners can seek to determine if their intervention had a significant effect on patient outcomes related to patient performance in activities of daily living and instrumental activities of daily living. The OBQI evidence can then be used to implement new care practices that may result in more favorable patient outcomes and ideally promote the value of occupational therapy.

The following resources offer information about OBQI:

- Home Health Agency (HHA) Center: www.cms.hhs.gov/center/hha.asp
- Colorado Health Outcomes Program, University of Colorado, Denver: www.uchsc.edu/coho

Using evidence—information that offers the patient, the third-party payer, and the physician an appreciation of the value of occupational therapy—is vital in the effort to promote the profession through best practice. When working with individuals in the home, occupational therapists and occupational therapy assistants are challenged to utilize the most current body of knowledge and empirical evidence to support what they are doing with their patients. This is not to diminish the importance and value of being able to think on your feet, of the skillfulness involved in therapeutic-use-of-self, and of the art of occupational therapy practice. The tacit knowledge that occupational therapy practitioners use in daily practice contributes to the success of treatment. In complement, using an evidence-based approach to design and implement intervention provides the practitioner with data to support the therapeutic benefits.

Documenting Skilled Service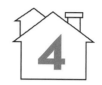

Karen Vance, OTR/L

ocumentation gives us the opportunity to create a picture not only of our patients but also of our profession. Documentation of our practice serves as a historical record for occupational therapy's contribution to any health care setting. Considering home health's history of occupational therapy underutilization, discussed in Chapter 2, the shift to outcome-focused quality monitoring presents a ripe environment for occupational therapy contribution to the home health setting. Even as these opportunities emerge, the principles of sound documentation presented here should remain constant. Focusing on three areas—target audience, clinical reasoning, and outcomes—will enable you to clearly and effectively describe your patient and your profession.

Who Is Your Target Audience?

Robertson (1998) described the various target audiences to consider when documenting service delivery. The target audience will influence what information you document and how you present it. In home health practice, the primary target audiences are *practitioners,* the *home health agency,* the *legal system, regulatory and accrediting agencies,* and *third-party payers.*

The authors express their gratitude to Mary Jo McGuire for her work on this chapter in the previous edition.

Practitioners

Practitioners document so they can maintain focused and effective intervention. Documentation serves to

- ensure comprehensive data collection,
- enable careful consideration of the patient's priorities and concerns,
- facilitate analysis of the diagnosis and care plan,
- focus on appropriate goals and plans of care,
- recall methods and media used,
- record communication and care coordination with the physician and other disciplines,
- describe the patient's response and contribution to the plan of care, and
- document when a patient has accomplished his or her goals.

Accurate documentation is critical to inform the best care planning and implementation. The medical record should clearly present the clinical reasoning that supports the need for occupational therapy and should describe the outcomes achieved as a result of occupational therapy.

If you are an occupational therapist (OTR) who is providing both evaluation and care, *you* are the practitioner audience for your own documentation. Therefore you need to provide only enough information about the visit to maintain continuity of care. A common pitfall is to write a detailed description of exactly what occurred during a visit. In fact, there is no need to record excessive treatment trivia in the medical record. Other target audiences are not interested in the minute details of your visit. The challenge is to summarize the visit in a way that substantiates effective clinical reasoning and clearly outlines plans for continued movement toward the targeted outcomes.

If you are evaluating patients and establishing a care plan that will be implemented by a certified occupational therapy assistant (COTA), the care plan must be documented in greater detail than is necessary when you are the care provider. The background and professional experience of the service provider will determine the amount of care plan information that must be documented. OTRs and COTAs have a joint responsibility to work as a team and maintain ongoing communication.

The Home Health Agency

It is also essential to document interdisciplinary communication. Logging communication provides evidence that practitioners are working to ensure efficient and comprehensive intervention. How interdisciplinary communication is documented varies according to the policies of the home health agency. No matter where communication is documented, you need to be certain to document not only formal team meetings but also every communication during which a patient's plan of care is discussed. Record the date and time, the topic of the discussion, and any issues related to the care plan or targeted outcome.

The home health agency through which occupational therapy is provided is a critical target audience and stakeholder in how occupational therapy service is delivered and documented because of the agency's reported outcomes. The public, the marketplace, and the Centers for Medicare and Medicaid Services (CMS) are all making decisions based on the outcomes reported by home health agencies, from choosing a home health agency to paying incentives for the best outcomes. Therefore it is paramount that documentation correlates the results achieved by occupational therapy services with the agency's outcomes.

The Legal System

With respect to legal considerations, Ranke (1998) advised always documenting both the date and the time of all communication between team members. Recording exactly when care is provided is standard practice, but documenting the exact time when communication with other professionals occurs may be a new habit. The note should be marked with the date when it is written, but it may reference services or observations made earlier. Ranke recommended that you never backdate or try to squeeze additional information into an existing notation; such actions may be construed as a cover-up attempt when placed under the scrutiny of the legal system. However, clearly dating and initialing a late entry on the same document is legal, acceptable, and a practical way to record additional information without excess pieces of paper. Corrections are made with a single strike-through line, ensuring the correction is initialed and dated at the time of correction.

Regulatory and Accrediting Agencies

The Medicare conditions of participation (CoPs) are the federal regulations that govern the basic quality standards required for every Medicare-certified home health agency (HHA). Unlike the coverage criteria required by Medicare as a payer for Medicare home health beneficiaries, the CoPs apply to all patients served by the HHA, regardless of payer source. They are the minimum quality *conditions* an agency must meet to *participate* in the Medicare program and are published in the *Federal Register* (CMS, 1999).

The Joint Commission on Accreditation of Healthcare Organizations (JCAHO), a consumer-oriented accrediting body, is the main accreditation target audience for home health. The JCAHO traditionally uses the practice standards established by each profession to evaluate the quality of care provided in that discipline (Siebert, 1997b). Therefore the American Occupational Therapy Association (AOTA) guidelines constitute the standard that the JCAHO uses to measure the quality of occupational therapy services. Home health agencies that are accredited or seeking accreditation should have a manual available for practitioners to review.

Most agencies use regulatory and accreditation standards as guidelines by which agency policies and procedures are written. Documentation and practice that comply with agency policies and procedures typically will in turn comply with federal regulations and quality accreditation standards.

Third-Party Payers

Because Medicare is the largest third-party payer in the United States, the expectations of many insurance companies parallel Medicare policies and regulations. Despite reimbursement changes, the coverage guidelines for occupational therapy in home health have not changed significantly since originally written. Current coverage guidelines are summarized in Chapter 2 and can be accessed at www.cms.hhs.gov/manuals; also refer to Appendix B for other resources.

References to federal documents are intended not to delimit the practice of occupational therapy but to assist you in addressing the concerns of the third-party payer as a target audience and ensuring accurate reimbursement to your home health agency.

Outcome and Assessment Information Set Versus Occupational Therapy Practice Framework

The CoPs for home health require a comprehensive assessment on all patients and the *Outcome and Assessment Information Set* (OASIS) (Shaughnessy, Crisler, Schlenker, & Hittle, 1998) integrated into the comprehensive assessment. As of this printing, the OASIS data collection and transmission requirement has been temporarily suspended for all but Medicare and Medicaid patients until further notice; however, many agencies have chosen to continue collecting data on all home health patients. The OASIS data set is intended to collect specific information at designated time points for measurement of outcomes. Any discussion of documentation in home care would be incomplete without a reference to it. According to the summary of regulations published by the CMS,

> The CoPs require that each patient receive from the HHA a patient-specific, comprehensive assessment that identifies the patient's medical, nursing, rehabilitative, social, and discharge planning needs. In addition, this rule requires that, as part of the comprehensive assessment, HHAs use a standard core assessment data set, the "Outcome and Assessment Information Set" (OASIS), when evaluating adult, non-maternity patients receiving skilled services other than homemaker or chore services only. This outcome data collection is an integral part of CMS' effort to achieve broad-based improvements in the quality of care furnished through Federal programs and in the measurement of that care. (CMS, 1999, p. 3764)

Though the outcome focus of these changes increases the opportunity for occupational therapy contribution, Medicare documents are not a primary source for understanding occupational therapy's domain of practice. The *Occupational Therapy Practice Framework* (AOTA, 2002c; henceforth *Framework*) outlines the domain of practice for the occupational therapy discipline. Table 4.1 compares performance outlined in the *Framework* with performance included in the OASIS. (OASIS item numbers are given in square brackets following the OASIS categories.) The OASIS covers most of the *Framework* activities describing activities of daily living (ADL) and instrumental activities of daily living (IADL)

TABLE 4.1
Comparison of *Occupational Therapy Practice Framework* and *Outcome and Assessment Information Set* (OASIS)

Occupational Therapy Practice Framework	OASIS data elements
Activities of daily living (area of occupation)	
Bathing, showering	Bathing [M0670]
Bowel and bladder management	Urinary incontinence presence [M0520] Urinary incontinence timing [M0530] Bowel incontinence frequency [M0540]
Dressing	Dressing upper body [M0650] Dressing lower body [M0660]
Eating, feeding	Feeding or eating [M0710]
Functional mobility	Toileting [M0680] (to and from only) Transferring [M0690] Ambulation/locomotion [M0700]
Personal device care	No equivalent
Personal hygiene and grooming	Grooming [M0640]
Sexual activity	No equivalent
Sleep, rest	No equivalent
Toilet hygiene	No equivalent
Instrumental activities of daily living (area of occupation)	
Care of others and pets	No equivalent
Child rearing	No equivalent
Communication device use	Ability to use telephone [M0770]
Community mobility	Transportation [M0730]
Financial management	No equivalent
Health management and maintenance	Management of oral meds [M0780] Management of inhalant/mist [M0790] Management of injectable meds [M0800]
Home establishment and management	Housekeeping [M0750] Laundry [M0740]
Meal preparation and cleanup	Planning/preparing light meals [M0720]
Safety procedures and emergency response	No equivalent
Shopping	Shopping [M0760]

areas of occupation; however, there are important distinctions between the OASIS and the *Framework*, including outcome definition and the increments of change.

The first distinction is the difference in how the two sources define outcomes. OASIS outcomes are defined as a change in the patient's health status between two or more time points (Shaughnessy et al., 1998). Because the OASIS measure is a data collection tool comparing the same data on all patients, the changes in the health status being measured must be consistent and specifically defined.

The *Framework* defines outcomes as important dimensions of health that are attributed to interventions, including ability to function, health perceptions, and satisfaction with care. The *Framework* describes the profession's overarching targeted outcome as "engagement in occupation to support participation" (AOTA, 2002c). Inherent in the client-centered nature of this definition is that the specific targeted outcome must be meaningful and purposeful to the patient. This distinction can be summarized as the difference between standardized outcomes and patient-defined outcomes.

The second distinction between the OASIS and the *Framework* is how increments of change in the patient's health status or health dimensions are measured. The OASIS levels of change span broader increments than *Framework*-guided documentation because the changes captured in OASIS data are measuring only the type and amount of assistance required for a patient to safely remain in his or her own home.

Framework-guided documentation can describe changes as detailed as those at a body function or body structure level and changes in the amount of assistance required for patient-specific occupational performance. Awareness of this distinction is important to prevent attempts at direct comparisons between the two measures. Using the *Framework* to document changes in the patient's health dimensions as a result of occupational therapy intervention is critical to expand the picture of the patient, as well as the picture of occupational therapy.

Documentation Format for Clinical Reasoning

The documentation format will either enable or restrict comprehensive care planning. Electronic or paper documentation packages purchased or developed by home health agencies will often dictate format. The home health clinician can either attempt to influence the format by participating in the agency's decision-making process for such packages or design a structure to link one's own clinical reasoning with the mandated documentation. Using the *Framework* to guide the process of evaluation, intervention, and outcome can guide how an occupational therapist organizes and documents clinical reasoning.

The evaluation process begins with the occupational therapist finding out what the patient wants and needs to do, because the overarching outcome is engagement in occupation to support participation in that which is meaningful to the patient. Therefore documentation is best led first by information gathered according to the *Framework*'s occupational profile: patient's occupational history and experiences, patterns of daily living, interests, values, and needs. Information obtained from the patient directs the analysis of occupational performance to identify the patient's assets, problems, or potential problems, which is the second step of the evaluation.

The documentation format should then lead to describing the patient's observed abilities during ADL, IADL, leisure, and social participation. Because performance skills (motor skills, process skills) and patterns (habits, routines, roles) used in occupational performance are identified during this analysis, they would be described next, followed by other aspects of engaging in occupation that affect skills and patterns such as context, activity demands, and patient factors (body functions, body structures). The *Framework* provides an excellent standard to ensure that documentation formatting is broad enough for use with all patients yet specific enough to cover each patient's particular concerns.

Evaluation

An evaluation can paint a picture of a patient, but the unique approach of occupational therapy frames the picture and projects an image of the profession. *Framework*-guided documentation can facilitate the individual occupational therapy process, but it can also explicitly describe the client-centered nature of the occupational therapy profession. Here is the first opportunity to document to multiple audiences: document first for the practitioner's clinical reasoning and then draw the connection for other stakeholders.

Remembering the difference in outcome definitions between the *Framework* and the OASIS, the occupational therapist structures the evaluation first by patient priorities that are internally motivated and individually defined and that require active participation by the patient. The *occupational profile* is a client-centered approach to understanding what is important and meaningful to the patient and identifying past experiences and interests that may assist problem solving and more efficiently guide interventions (AOTA, 2002c). Gathering the patient's occupational history not only informs a better intervention plan but also allows the occupational therapist to describe the patient's prior functional status, which is typically sought by external audiences, particularly payers.

Consider the following example: The patient is a 73-year-old grandmother who complains that it wears her out to cook a full meal and be around the grandkids and that it takes her too long to prepare to leave the house. She is a widow of 10 years who has "always taken care of herself" and has always "done Thanksgiving" for her two children and five grandchildren, who live nearby. Until recently, she lived alone independently and occasionally drove short distances.

The occupational profile uncovers some of the roles and routines that help narrow the occupational performances specific to this patient. Then the *analysis of occupational performance* identifies the current performance skills and patterns used in the patient's occupational performance, as well as other factors such as body functions, activity demands, and contexts that affect performance (AOTA, 2002c). The *Framework* describes selecting specific assessments to measure performance and other factors as part of the analysis process. Selecting industry-specific measures is also another opportunity to speak to other stakeholder audiences.

The occupational therapist can satisfy several stakeholders by drawing the connection between the performances measured by the occupational therapist and the outcome indicators recorded on the OASIS. Though it is outside the scope of this manual to provide specific training on OASIS data collection, we highly recommend that all home health practitioners maintain proficiency in understanding each OASIS data element, the specific response items within each data element, and the special instructions provided in the OASIS user's manual (www. cms.gov/oasis). Table 4.1 compares areas addressed in the *Framework* with OASIS outcome indicators, but it does not reveal how specifically each response item is worded to standardize each increment of change to increase the interrater reliability of the OASIS data collection set. For example, an occupational therapist may observe a patient don and doff usual clothing and document the patient as independent in dressing. However, the OASIS items of upper and lower body dressing include obtaining the items from closets or drawers. Including this performance in measuring and documenting dressing would give more specific and relevant information to the home health agency.

Remember that the levels of change between the OASIS responses do not reflect the more sensitive increments measured by an occupational therapy evaluation. Historically, rehabilitation professionals have used measurements once published in the *Medicare Outpatient Physical Therapy and Comprehensive Outpatient Rehabilitation Manual* (hereafter shortened to *Medicare Outpatient Manual*) (Health Care Financing Administration [HCFA], 1998). The detailed descriptors for this 6-point scale provide a much more sensitive instrument for measuring progress. (More information on the use of scales can be found in the "Documenting for Medicare" section in this chapter.) It is important to provide these measurable and objective increments to provide a good baseline picture for developing reasonable and measurable goals and interventions.

Goals or Targeted Outcomes

Establishing appropriate goals is an opportunity for OTRs to satisfy multiple stakeholders: the patient, the payer, the home health agency, and, most important, the profession. Beginning with the occupational profile, the OTR can ascertain the patient's priorities and desired targeted outcomes, which is critical to establishing the appropriateness of goals and useful for identifying a meaningful, occupation-based plan of care. A plan of care that is driven by the patient's targeted outcomes is one in which the patient is more likely to take ownership. Patient self-management is the ultimate goal of every home health plan of care, regardless of diagnosis or eventual desired occupational performance. The advantage in the home health setting is that the home is the very context where the patient will be performing the achieved goals. The challenge is to empower the patient to manage his or her own health and to sustain or continue pursuing goals after the intervention is completed.

Establishing reasonable, measurable, and objective goals for a relevant time span is also critical for communicating to the payer the value of the treatment plan for the resources being compensated. The time span relevant to home health is the certification period covered by the plan of care. Because Medicare's time frame is limited to 60 days, it is necessary to identify the performance expected at the end of the 60 days, with a broader goal defined that may be achieved in subsequent episodes of care. Estimating time points when outcomes may be achieved communicates reasonable expectations for the frequency and duration of the plan of care. Well-written goals will also make it easier to demonstrate the effectiveness of the plan of care and the contribution by occupational therapy in achieving the outcomes.

Using language that correlates goals to the outcomes identified in the OASIS will help the home health agency easily extract data for record review and the outcome-based quality improvement (OBQI) process. Even though occupational therapists may document smaller increments of change than the OASIS measures, goals similarly worded to the increments of change captured on the OASIS will assist the agency in identifying whether certain OASIS outcomes have improved, stabilized, or declined: for example, write "Patient will complete grooming and dressing independently and within usual time frame without shortness of breath" when addressing energy conservation for a patient with congestive heart failure. Also, because the OASIS item that addresses toileting refers only to whether the patient can safely access the toilet, an OTR will want to identify the aspects of toileting addressed in a goal, such as "Patient will be independent in manipulating clothing with assistive devices to use the bedside commode" rather than just "Patient will be independent in toileting." A correlation to OASIS-defined outcomes assists the profession because it demonstrates to the home health agency how valuable occupational therapy is in achieving desired outcomes.

Outcome Stabilization

In cases where realistic expectations for improvement in performance areas cannot be identified, OTRs may be able to support the value in the stabilization of outcomes to prevent deterioration or compromised safety. The prevalence of chronic, long-term conditions in the home health patient population warrants stabilization as a desirable outcome and requires a reevaluation of occupational therapy clinical reasoning and practice patterns. "Instead of considering the potential for improvement with occupational therapy, the therapist must evaluate the patient's potential for declining performance without occupational therapy" (Vance & Siebert, 2007, p. CE-4). Particularly with the emphasis from the CMS to decrease the rate of acute care hospitalization, stabilization for chronic patients can be more than the absence of a negative outcome, if stabilization actually improves an agency's hospitalization rate.

Plan of Care

The plan of care (POC) is the intervention plan to be carried out by the OTR and COTA. POC development is based on findings from the evaluation and driven by the identified goals or targeted outcomes. The occupational therapy plan is part of an agency POC required by the CoPs, and for Medicare it is the Home Health Certification and Plan of Care, or Form 485, as described in Chapter 2. For the practitioner audience who will be carrying out the POC, the interventions should be documented with a level of detail that can be followed by the COTA or substitute therapist. Developing a POC to meet the expectations of other audiences requires knowledge of those specifically required elements.

The POC is a legal document and must be signed by the physician. Certain elements are required by Medicare coverage guidelines to be present on the POC for each discipline:

- pertinent diagnoses or conditions being treated,
- skilled interventions that are reasonable and necessary for the diagnosis or condition,
- frequency and duration reasonable for the diagnosis or condition,
- goals reflecting services planned with reasonable time estimates for completion,
- date the order was received, and
- date the order is effective.

The specific occupational therapy POC may be included on Form 485 or documented on a supplemental order to Form 485, or in some agencies the completed evaluation is sent to the physician for the signature and returned to the agency. Whether or not the occupational therapy plan is included on Form 485, it is a legal order, and evidence that the orders are followed must be in the visit documentation. So the level of detail in the intervention plan should allow for some flexibility on a visit-by-visit basis.

Visit Notes

The practitioner documents a record of services after every visit. As mentioned during the discussion of documentation format, most agencies have visit forms or electronic documentation that may dictate how the visit is documented. However, the goals or performance areas and underlying deficits identified in the evaluation can structure the clinical reasoning behind documenting for the various target audiences.

Leading the visit note with goals and performance areas assists the practitioner to focus on movement toward the targeted outcome, followed by interventions outlined from the plan of care designed to achieve the targeted outcomes. For the OTR–COTA team, this sequence provides a map to ensure the intervention continues to be appropriate. Though the intervention may be addressing performance skills or a body function, relating the intervention back to the desired performance area helps the therapist maintain an occupation-based approach.

The agency as an audience also benefits on two counts from documentation that relates the intervention back to desired performance areas: (a) during the episode of care, team members have a clear understanding of what occupational therapy is doing on the plan of care, and (b) it makes for easier chart review later, especially for the OBQI process of care investigation.

The legal system, quality accreditors, and third-party payers also require certain elements to be present in each visit note. As noted earlier, the visit note provides evidence that the orders are being followed. Documenting for quality accreditors includes providing elements that prove compliance with policies, regulations, and quality standards. Also include the elements required to satisfy the third-party payers that coverage criteria are met. For Medicare, the largest payer, that includes evidence of skilled service, homebound status, and sufficient progress toward stated goals.

Documenting for Medicare

Skilled therapy services must be reasonable and necessary to the treatment of the patient's illness or injury within the context of the patient's unique medical condition. For services to be considered reasonable and necessary, the following conditions must be met:

1. The services must be consistent with the nature and severity of the illness or injury and the patient's particular medical needs.

2. The services must be specific, safe, and effective treatment for the patient's condition, under accepted standards of medical practice.

3. The services must be provided with the expectation, based on the assessment of the patient's rehabilitation potential made by the physician, that the condition of the patient will improve materially in a reasonable and generally predictable period of time or that the services are necessary to the establishment of a safe and effective maintenance program. (The term *materially* means having real importance to consequences and to an important degree, or the improvement can be perceived in material form [objectively]. In general, there should be a reasonable expectation that observable improvement in the overall safety of functional ability will occur.)

4. Services of skilled therapists for the purpose of teaching the patient or the patient's family or caregivers necessary techniques, exercises, or precautions are covered to the extent that they are reasonable and necessary to treat illness or injury.

5. The amount, frequency, and duration of the services must be reasonable.

The Cahaba Government Benefit Administrators' *Coverage Guidelines for Home Health Agencies* (2006) lists examples of documentation showing measurable improvement that could include one or more of the following areas:

• *Change of one assistance grade (level):* The beneficiary has advanced from minimum assist to supervised with verbal cueing in upper body dressing. The levels are defined as maximum, minimum, standby (supervised), and independent.

- *Increased consistency:* The documentation reveals that the beneficiary responds by inconsistently performing functional tasks from day to day or within a treatment session. Increased consistency within the same level of assistance may reflect improvement.

  Patients may show signs of progress by beginning to recall the sequence of a compensatory method or by self-correcting when they begin to perform an activity unsafely. Consistency is necessary for the development of safe habits. Documenting when a patient is inconsistent in performing safely or independently enables you to record improvement when consistency increases.

- *Increased generalization:* The beneficiary is able to apply concepts and performance previously learned in one activity to another similar activity.

  The occupational adaptation frame of reference (Schkade & Schultz, 1992; Schultz & Schkade, 1992) provides a strong theoretical foundation for the critical role of generalization in the process of adaptation. The process of adaptation requires people to explore and attempt new activities. Therefore a patient's effort to try a new activity or method outside of therapy is evidence that the process of adaptation is occurring. The effects of direct care can often be seen during nontherapy time when a patient musters the courage and energy to attempt a new activity. This is great news for home care practitioners who arrive at a patient's home prepared to engage the patient in an activity only to discover that the patient has already attempted (and perhaps mastered) it. Generalization is evidence of progress. Practitioners should document the skilled observation that the patient's behavior between visits demonstrates generalization.

- *New functional activity initiated:* This might consist of adding lower body dressing following a program of upper body dressing.

Do not gloss over the incorporation of a new task into the treatment regime, because this is another sign of progress. Moreover, the documentation of a plan to do an actual performance assessment constitutes evidence of the need for skilled services.

- *New compensatory technique (with or without equipment) added:* This might consist of teaching the beneficiary the use of a stocking aide for lower body dressing.

Each time you present a modified or adapted method, make a recommendation to adjust a compensatory method, or plan to incorporate a new therapeutic strategy to increase safety or independence, progress is made. Carefully monitor your own behavior so you can document this type of progress.

Change in Level of Assistance

The *Medicare Outpatient Manual* (HCFA, 1998b) provides a 6-point scale with detailed physical and cognitive descriptors for use in rating a patient's level of independence in performance areas. The following outline is excerpted from the document:

1. Total assistance
   a. Minimal voluntary motor actions
   b. 100% assistance from one or more helpers
2. Maximum assistance
   a. 75% assistance from one person
   b. Physical support with each step
   c. One-on-one demonstration
3. Moderate assistance
   a. 50% assistance
   b. Assistance every time activity is performed
   c. Intermittent demonstration
   d. Occupational therapist or caregiver in immediate area
4. Minimal assistance
   a. 25% assistance
   b. Provide setup assistance
   c. Help to initiate or sustain an activity

    d. Review of alternate procedures, sequences, and methods

    e. Reminders to correct repeated mistakes

    f. Check of compliance regarding safety

    g. Assistance to solve problems posed by unexpected hazard

5. Standby assistance

    a. Supervision in using adaptive methods

    b. Safety precautions

6. Independent status

    a. Neither assistance nor supervision

A comparative analysis of these descriptors with the terminology commonly used in occupational therapy reveals several discrepancies. For instance, the Medicare descriptors do not provide for "moderate assistance of two"; if two helpers are necessary, the patient needs total assistance under the Medicare guidelines. Many practitioners confess that they habitually rate patients as needing less assistance than a strict use of the CMS's descriptors would warrant. For example, the first time a patient is introduced to a piece of adaptive equipment, practitioners often provide one-on-one demonstration of safe and appropriate use. Most practitioners would document this as minimal or moderate assistance, whereas it is rated as maximum assistance on the CMS scale. Applying the more stringent standard, however, allows leeway for demonstrating progress. Using a scale at least as sensitive as the CMS scale allows you to report the small steps of progress toward goals.

Choose one level of assistance when rating a patient, avoiding double-level reporting, such as "min-mod" or "mod-max." It is wise to rate patients who are between levels at the lower level and document that the person is "inconsistently able to perform at the higher level." For example, "Mr. R. requires moderate assistance for lower extremity dressing but is inconsistently able to perform with minimal assistance."

The services of skilled therapists for the purpose of teaching the patient or the patient's family or caregivers necessary techniques, exercises, or precautions are covered to the extent that they are reasonable and necessary to treat illness or injury. The learner's response to any instruction—that is, what is inadequate in the learner's performance—is critical information to document. One way to identify these inadequacies is to monitor your own behavior during the instruction, asking yourself questions such as these:

- When and why do I intervene?
- What cues or comments do I offer during the return demonstration?

This type of self-monitoring will provide the content to document the need for continued instruction. The following examples support the need for continued instruction:

- Mr. R. required cues to properly pace himself to avoid falling.
- Mrs. L.'s husband had difficulty handling her left upper extremity during passive range of motion; he needed cues to move her limb at the proper speed to avoid eliciting a stretch reflex.
- Mr. J. is not able to recall the proper sequence of steps to don his clothing using compensatory techniques.
- Ms. S. needs step-by-step cueing to safely transfer from her wheelchair to the tub bench.

The following example illustrates how the need for continued instruction should be professionally documented:

> *Dressing:* The occupational therapist evaluated the effectiveness of compensatory methods demonstrated last session. Methods were modified to increase safety; patient inconsistently remembered the proper movement sequence needed for donning her blouse.

Following instruction, and even during an active care plan, you may need to write in lay terms specific instructions or recommendations to the patient or caregiver and reference them in the medical record. Always retain duplicates of such written information in your records for reference, but they do not necessarily have to be filed in the medical record. You must be able to produce evidence of the exact recommendations or maintenance program provided to a patient or caregiver. You are responsible for determining what information you place in the medical record (target audience: team members, third-party payers, legal system) and what you give to the patient or family and maintain in your own records (target audience: you, patient or family, and legal system or third-party payer if more information is required on appeal).

When skilled services relate to adaptive equipment or environmental modifications, always document your recommendations and the patient's or caregiver's response. This principle is equally important whether the patient accepts or rejects the recommendation. Documenting the patient's or caregiver's rejection of a recommendation may protect you from legal repercussions if an injury occurs after the patient is discharged.

Document skilled services in which meaningful occupations are used to develop performance skills according to the needs of the target audience. Too much emphasis on the details of the activity demands can camouflage the therapeutic nature of the session. The challenge is to summarize the therapeutic principles or strategies incorporated into common ADL (see Table 4.2 for examples).

Describing Underlying Performance Skill and Performance Pattern Deficits

An important aspect of skilled occupational therapy services is ongoing analysis of the relationship of performance skills and patterns to performance areas; that is, which motor, process, and communication and interaction skills and habits, routines, or roles are interfering with the patient's ability to perform relevant areas of occupation. The medical necessity of occupational therapy intervention is demonstrated through clear articulation of the underlying factors that prevent an individual from safely or independently engaging in an activity. Clearly state the relationship between impairments and function so that reviewers do not have to analyze raw data or draw conclusions based on extensive detail (see Table 4.3 for examples).

Discharge Notes

A patient may be discharged from home care for several reasons. Three of the major reasons are (a) the goals have been accomplished and the patient is self-managing, (b) sufficient progress has been made so the patient is no longer homebound, and (c) the patient is rehospitalized

TABLE 4.2
Emphasizing the Therapeutic Nature of Activities of Daily Living

Occupation and context	Performance skill correlation[a]
Mrs. L. removed clothes from the clothes dryer while sitting on a chair.	Energy conservation: Mrs. L. engaged in a homemaking activity from a sitting position and was instructed in energy conservation skills.
Mr. D. prepared a simple cold meal with a hot beverage for lunch. He needed cues to visually scan his environment to find the needed objects.	Visual attention: Mr. D. participated in simple cold meal prep and was instructed in visual scanning techniques and safety awareness.
Mrs. K. retrieved her clothes from her bedroom closet and laid them on the bed prior to her shower.	Range of motion, endurance, balance, mobility: Mrs. K. engaged in activities of daily living to increase left upper extremity range of motion, endurance, and dynamic balance.
The occupational therapist instructed Mrs. K. in shower transfers. Mrs. K. completed a shower and got dressed. Mrs. K. asked for assistance to reach her legs to get dressed.	Safety awareness, mobility: Mrs. K. completed a sitting transfer with supervision and good safety awareness. Mrs. K. completed upper extremity dressing independently and lower extremity dressing with minimal assistance.

[a]These are excerpts, not complete daily visit notes.

because of medical instability. Regardless of the reason for discharge, a discharge note must be written. The simplest format is to organize the note by the goals established for the patient. A useful discharge note provides a list of the goals, a record of whether each goal was accomplished or partially met, the patient's status at the beginning of the program, the therapeutic methods and media used, and the patient's status at discharge. Also be certain to retain clear records of any home program or functional maintenance program that was established during care.

TABLE 4.3
Documenting Outcomes

Reporting of events or skills	Documenting outcomes
Mrs. L. continually gets short of breath during meal preparation (chronic obstructive pulmonary disease). She does not stop to rest. She reports she "just needs to get it done."	Mrs. L. was instructed in energy conservation techniques during kitchen activities. Using these techniques allows her to prepare a simple meal without getting short of breath.
Mr. K. does not take his medication adequately to prevent low blood sugar levels, resulting in frequent falls (diabetes).	Mr. K. was assisted in relocating his medication to match his temporal routine. He has improved consistency in accurately taking his medications.
Mr. T. sits in front of the TV the majority of the day. He is unable to tolerate more than 15 minutes of activity at one time (congestive heart failure).	Mr. T. was instructed and participated in upper extremity endurance activities, which allowed him to safely complete a shower with supervision in 30 minutes.

Conclusion

Thoughtful and thorough documentation reflects an accurate picture of the individual patient, reflects the profession, and provides an opportunity for a personal reflection of your own practice. The core purpose of occupational therapy services is to accomplish the patient's goals or targeted outcomes. Outcome-oriented practice is best reflected in outcome-oriented documentation. If you work with your patients in establishing and achieving reasonable goals, you will find that documentation supports your work. It keeps you focused and becomes a platform on which the effectiveness of intervention is displayed. Identify reasonable goals and document the effectiveness of your therapy in achieving outcomes for all audiences.

The Clinic Called *Home* 5

Carol Siebert, MS, OTR/L, FAOTA

Practice in the home presents challenges and opportunities like no other venue for occupational therapy services. It offers the occupational therapy practitioner an opportunity to enter the context of a patient's life and to provide intervention in the environment that most intimately reflects the patient's values, roles, and personality. That context also presents more significant and more intense challenges than do other settings, because community, architecture, finances, and family interactions, as well as payment and public policy, affect the services the practitioner provides in the home. The word *clinic* connotes a place where the practitioner is in charge and there is order and regularity. The home is a much more dynamic and complex setting for occupational therapy than any clinic.

This chapter explores the practicalities of providing occupational therapy in the home and how this practice is different from practice in a clinic. The first section establishes the context for 21st-century home health practice. The next section explores the dynamics of home care practice and the relationship with the patient. This section also addresses the challenges created by the physical, social, and cultural environment. The meanings of home and of facing disablement in the home are also discussed. The next section establishes a framework for coherent assessment and intervention to address the complexities of context, caregivers, and patient priorities in home care. Constructs from the *International Classification of Function, Disability and Health* (World Health Organization [WHO], 2001), the *Occupational Therapy Practice Framework* (American Occupational Therapy Association [AOTA], 2002c), and the *Person–Environment–Occupation Model* (Law et al., 1996) are introduced in this section and are integrated throughout the remainder of the chapter.

The next section addresses intervention, including strategies to optimize both home visits and the interval between visits. This section also covers two unique aspects of intervention in home care: making environmental modifications and working with caregivers. The physical environment plays a much more significant role in home care than in other practice settings. The home environment has a direct impact on the outcomes that can be achieved through occupational therapy and an impact on safety. Home care practice involves untrained caregivers, typically family members, who have an emotional and financial stake in the outcome achieved through occupational therapy. The discussion includes issues such as establishing shared expectations with caregivers, teaching caregivers, and managing your role as a professional when dealing with family dynamics.

The final section explores the perceptions and experiences of the patient as intervention proceeds in the home. Satisfaction and competence are addressed. This section explores the psychosocial practice skills needed in home care, as the importance of *meaning* in home care. A case study illustrates some of the principles discussed in this chapter.

The Larger Context of Home Health

Home health practice is based on the Medicare home health benefit. This is because Medicare regulations govern all services provided by home health agencies and also because Medicare is the dominant payer for home health care. (Refer to Chapter 2 for a detailed explanation.) Patients must be homebound to receive home health services under Medicare Part A and most other payers. Thus, home health patients often have complex health problems or significant functional limitations that render them homebound. Most home health patients are older adults or adults with disabling conditions. The reason for referral to home care may be a new onset of a condition or an exacerbation of an existing condition or conditions. A small number of home health referrals are for patients with no previous health problems to address short-term, resolvable health conditions. However, it is more common to encounter patients who are older, have multiple health conditions, have one or more functional limitations, and have experienced a decline in health and function over a period of months or years. These are individuals who are at risk of being unable to adequately manage their health and daily activities in their homes. They are at risk of having to obtain more intensive caregiving in the home or of having to move to secure additional caregiving, whether from a family member (moving in with relatives) or from an institutional setting (moving to an assisted living or nursing facility). Often the most important priority of the patient and the family is for the patient to be able to stay in the home. However, this expectation of home care is often unspoken.

For years, home health services, including occupational therapy services, were driven by regulations and payment requirements based on practice in inpatient or outpatient acute settings. Payment was based on the provision of a "skilled service"—a visit. The need for services was based on findings of clinical deficits or impairments. The need for therapy had to be supported by a potential for improvement in function, demonstrated by measurable changes in skills or body functions (e.g., range of motion, strength, level of task assistance). The result of these factors was that home health occupational therapy, provided to older homebound adults with deteriorating health and function and multiple chronic conditions, was little different from inpatient or outpatient occupational therapy provided to adults in acute rehab. For the most part, patients seen for home health occupational therapy were referred based on the same criteria (e.g., diagnosis, rehab potential) used in inpatient rehab.

Startling data yielded by the Medicare Home Health Quality Initiative (HHQI) (www.cms.hhs.gov/HomeHealthQualityInits/) challenge assumptions about care based on these premises. For several years, the number of home health patient episodes that end with the patient being discharged to the community has remained at 65% (Home Health Quality Improvement Support Center, 2007). This means that 35%—more than one in three—home health patients go to a hospital, nursing home, or other inpatient health care facility (not assisted living). The overall percentage of home health patients who have an acute hospitalization while receiving home health care has remained at 28% since 2004. The data suggest that home health services as they have been provided are failing to achieve the number one priority for most patients—to be able to manage in the home and remain at home.

These data are of interest to policy makers, because hospitalizations and transfers to institutional settings increase Medicare and Medicaid expenditures. Equally important, they indicate that the increased amount of public dollars spent is not producing a commensurate improvement in patient health and, in many cases, is failing to even stabilize patient health and function. As a result, a growing number of policy initiatives are focused on improving quality of care and linking payment to quality.

For years, home health occupational therapy practitioners have bemoaned payment and regulatory requirements that seemed at odds with occupational therapy's values and counterproductive to treating the whole person. But public policy—payment and regulation—is converging with patient priorities: expecting that home health services will enable patients to manage their health and daily activities to be able to remain at home. What this convergence means is that home health occupational therapy services must produce outcomes that matter to the clients: the patient and the payer. This expectation is completely consistent with occupational therapy values and traditions—and occupational therapy skills and expertise have never been more needed in home health. The rest of this chapter outlines perspectives, strategies, and tools for providing occupational therapy in home health that truly make a difference for patients and payers.

Therapy in Real Life

As a home health practitioner, you have a role not found in other settings of practice: you are a guest in the patient's home. From the first time you walk in the door, the patient and caregivers have expectations of you not only as a professional service provider but also as a visitor to their home. Some patients expect a very formal, professional relationship. Others treat any visitor as part of the family and expect you to be comfortable in that role. Seldom do patients verbalize these expectations, so you must follow their lead as to how the relationship will unfold.

These expectations about the relationship extend to issues such as how you and the patient address each other, how visits are scheduled, and what behavior is acceptable. Although these issues may occasionally arise in other settings, they are daily challenges in home care. When patients are on your turf, whether on an inpatient or outpatient basis, you have a tacit acknowledgment that the practitioner is in charge, and the patient has a responsibility to follow the rules and conventions of the facility. In those settings late sleepers can be roused by staff and escorted by patient transportation to arrive at the clinic promptly at 8:30 a.m. Patients, whether they are 25 or 85 years old, are routinely addressed by their first name by everyone from the physician to the orderly.

In the home the patient is in charge, and you must discern the expectations and conventions of each home we enter. Patients who prefer to sleep late may routinely decline appointments before noon or may not answer the door when callers arrive earlier. Patients may tolerate being called by their first name in the home, but other family members may be offended to hear the family matriarch or patriarch being addressed in such a manner by a stranger. Some patients will make home health services a priority and schedule other visitors around these appointments, whereas other patients may prioritize visits from clergy or family and change or cancel visits that conflict with these other interests. A patient who spends a lot of time alone may welcome the social contact you provide, agree to visits at any time, and press you to stay and chat. Other patients will be highly offended if you are not at the door within 5 minutes of the scheduled time. In home health, being "client centered" begins with the recognition that the patient has a life and that there are other activities and interests that are important to the patient. Although being in the home offers you cues to these other interests, it is easy to generalize a "clinic" mind-set and expect that therapy should be the patient's first priority. When working in the home, you must recognize the patient's priorities and determine what the patient expects of home health generally and occupational therapy specifically. It is possible to negotiate expectations but only after recognizing and respecting the priorities of the patient.

As mentioned earlier, being in the home means you are not on your own turf. It means that how you respond to and interact with those in the home and with the home itself is a factor that is not present in other practice settings. Some patients will give you the run of the house; these are often the same patients who treat you like a friend or family member. Other patients are more formal and expect you to ask permission to enter any room other than the one to which you have been escorted. Assessing the physical environment must be done in a manner that is acceptable to the patient. Some patients will be concerned about neatness and cleanliness and worry about offending you with an unmade bed or dirty dishes, whereas other patients may be entirely unconcerned about what you think of their home. It is wise to get to know the patient before making statements about the environment.

Other inhabitants or visitors in the home pose additional challenges. A patient may be willing to accommodate your scheduling needs and treatment plans, but a spouse may resent being disturbed by an early-morning visit. Other visitors or even family members may pose confidentiality challenges, as the patient may not wish them to know about his or her health or functional status. Especially challenging is the situation where you enter the home to find other individuals present who are not immediately introduced and who may be family, friends, or onetime visitors. In this case you must balance the "guest" and "professional" roles without compromising the patient's right to confidentiality.

Another challenge in the home is the ethical mandate to treat patients in an unbiased manner. When in a home you may be confronted by political, religious, and social viewpoints that are offensive or even provocative. Patients and their families may interact in ways that are normal and comfortable for them but uncomfortable for you. Conventions about how to talk to one's spouse or children or how to treat one's pets vary widely in our society. Patients may define "clean" (referring to either their house or their person) in ways that differ from your own perceptions. As a home care practitioner, you are frequently confronted with widely divergent values, opinions, and beliefs that may differ considerably from your own. You have a professional obligation to report situations where an individual is being neglected, abused, or exploited, but it is important to remain keenly aware that circumstances you find offensive or uncomfortable may be perfectly normal to that patient and family and that they would be embarrassed or offended by your opinion of the situation. There is also the risk of becoming too involved. It is essential to maintain professionalism and establish professional boundaries to avoid burnout from becoming immersed in complex life situations during every visit.

All of these issues mean that the moment you step in the door, home care presents challenges that are minimized or nonexistent in other treatment settings. Meeting these challenges is critical to success in home care. You might deliver high-quality, effective intervention and assist the patient to achieve functional outcomes, but if the patient or family perceives you as judgmental, bossy, biased, or condescending, that is what they will focus on and remember about the encounter. Several years ago a fieldwork student summed up this challenge by stating, "In home care you have to be a different person in every home you enter." This leads to a key question: Who does this patient need me to be for therapy to be effective? Reflecting on the question and operationalizing the answer will greatly influence effectiveness of therapy. Part of the art of home care is having the ability to be a professional and also be who the patient needs you to be.

The richness and complexity of therapy in context presents opportunities not encountered in other settings. Directly assessing an individual's performance in the home environment provides realistic and accurate information about his or her strengths and needs, as well as immediate feedback regarding the appropriateness and efficacy of intervention. The environment provides clues to what must be assessed. For example, if you must traverse a gravel walkway and climb eight steps to reach the front door of the home, the challenge of home access and egress for an individual in a wheelchair or with limited ambulation becomes obvious. Likewise, narrow or obstructed pathways, poor lighting, and loose doorknobs or towel racks can provide clues about fall hazards and how the patient has improvised solutions to these problems. The environment of the home may also indicate the reasons why a technique learned in a clinic may not generalize to the home. For example, bed mobility techniques learned on a hospital bed or on a mat table may be useless on a high bed with a worn-out mattress. Issues of environmental control (e.g., illumination, ventilation, and sanitation) that never arise in other settings become significant issues to assess in the home setting. These factors point to the need for dynamic assessment, not simply assessing the client and then the environment but assessing the client's actual performance in the environment.

Working with family and other informal caregivers presents unexpected challenges. In the familiar confines of their home, caregivers may voice frustrations or expectations regarding the patient that they would be hesitant to offer in other settings. Family dynamics are disrupted by role changes when the patient becomes the one cared for and other family members assume the caregiver role. You must adjust to working with caregivers whose level of knowledge, willingness, or cooperation may vary greatly. To complicate matters further, the schedule of caregiving may be such that the caregiver present during a therapy visit may not be the person who will actually implement the assistance strategies you wish to promote.

Along with the complexities of the physical, social, and cultural context, the role changes and losses experienced by the patient are another constant challenge in home care. While undergoing inpatient hospitalization or rehabilitation, the patient may anticipate home as being the place where things will be familiar, where everything will be all right. It is unfortunate that the return home is often very different. Familiar rooms and belongings can become alien and threatening when taken-for-granted abilities are affected by illness, injury, or disease. A favorite easy chair may become a symbol of defeat for a patient who can no longer rise from that chair except with assistance. The comfort of a familiar room may seem alien when a hospital bed and bedside commode arrive and cherished belongings are displaced by medical equipment, dressing supplies, or unpacked souvenirs of the inpatient stay. A bowling trophy or knitting prize may become a mocking reminder of lost skills when hemiplegia or arthritis makes even simple movements difficult or painful. This paradox of the familiar becoming threatening and alien is not uncommon when patients come home from an inpatient stay. Compensatory strategies that seemed a triumph in an inpatient setting may feel like giving in and giving up on improvement upon returning home (Wallenbert & Jonsson, 2005). Family members may bristle when the patient seems to sulk or resist participation in familiar activities, but often the patient is unable to articulate the feelings triggered by returning home. Especially for an older adult who has lived many years in one dwelling, the home is an extension and a reflection of the self. To feel out of place or powerless in one's own home may evoke deep feelings of helplessness and even hopelessness.

Clinical Thinking Tools

Daily living at home involves a myriad of activities embedded in a familiar environment and executed in manners and sequences that are unique to the individual or family. Basic activities of daily living (ADL)—bathing, dressing, toileting—are important but compose only a small portion of daily activities. The context, the physical environment, the meaning of activities, the experiences of the patient, and the expectations and assistance available from others affect performance in the home and thus figure prominently in assessment and intervention.

This complexity can seem overwhelming. There are three tools used in this section and the remainder of the chapter that provide terminology and provide a thinking frame for practice in the home. The tools are the *International Classification of Functioning, Disability and Health* (ICF; WHO, 2001), the *Occupational Therapy Practice Framework* (*Framework*; AOTA, 2002c), and the *Person–Environment–Occupation Model* (PEO; Law et al., 1996).

The ICF is an internationally recognized taxonomy. "The overall aim of the ICF . . . is to provide a unified and standard language and framework for the description of health and health-related states. It defines components of health and some health-related components of well-being" (WHO, 2001, p. 3). The ICF has two parts, each with two components. These are identified in Table 5.1.

The ICF distinguishes between *activity*—the execution of a task or action by an individual—and *participation*—the involvement in a life situation. *Activity limitations* are difficulties an individual may have in executing activities. *Participation restrictions* are problems an individual may experience in involvement in life situations (WHO, 2001, p. 12). ICF also distinguishes between *capacity* and *performance*. *Capacity* refers to "an individual's ability to execute a task or an action. This construct aims to indicate the highest probable level of functioning that a person may reach in a given domain at a given moment" (p. 15). In contrast, *performance* refers to "what an individual does in his or her current environment. Because the current environment includes a societal context, performance can also be understood as 'involvement in a life situation' or 'the lived experience' of people in the actual context in which they live. This context includes the environmental factors—all aspects of the physical, social and attitudinal world" (p. 15).

The distinction between capacity and performance points to one of the biggest differences between practice in the clinic and practice in the home. In a clinic setting, the patient's ability to execute a task occurs in a standard environment. Intervention focuses on improving skills and reducing the assistance needed to perform the task in that environment. Adaptive equipment may be used to enhance performance. Many assessment tools used in inpatient settings rate both the execution of each activity and the intensity of human and technological assistance.

TABLE 5.1

Selected Aspects of the International Classification of Functioning, Disability and Health (ICF)

	Part 1: Functioning and disability		Part 2: Contextual factors	
	Body functions and structures	Activities and participation	Environmental factors	Personal factors
Components	Body functions and structures	Activities and participation	Environmental factors	Personal factors
Domains	Body functions Body structures	Life areas (tasks, actions)	External influences on functioning and disability	Internal influences on functioning and disability
Constructs	Change in body functions (physiological) Change in body structures (anatomical)	Capacity: Executing tasks in a standard environment Performance: Executing tasks in the current environment	Facilitating or hindering impact of features of the physical, social, and attitudinal world	Impact of attributes of the person

Note. From International Classification of Functioning, Disability and Health (p. 11), by World Health Organization, 2001, Geneva, Switzerland. Copyright 2001 by the World Health Organization.

Interventions are directed toward improving the ratings. This is an assessment of *capacity*. In the inpatient environment, assistance and support are always available to ensure that personal care and environmental management is completed regardless of the patient's ability to execute these tasks.

In the home, the physical environment bears little similarity to the clinic, increasing task complexity. Family caregivers may be unable or unwilling to provide intensive round-the-clock assistance that is taken for granted in an inpatient setting. Assessment, and thus intervention, must be directed toward performance and participation: *the patient's daily engagement in activities in the social and physical environment of the home.*[1]

The *Occupational Therapy Practice Framework* (AOTA, 2002c) articulates the *domain* and *process* of occupational therapy. One of the stated purposes of the *Framework* is "to describe the domain that centers and grounds the profession's focus and actions" (p. 609). Some of the constructs of the domain are derived from the ICF. Other constructs have no correlates in the ICF but capture important aspects of performance. These include performance patterns (roles, habits, routines) and activity demands.

Occupational therapy has a long history of valuing the rhythm and patterns of activities: habits and routines. In clinical settings, tasks are performed according to schedules established to meet the efficiency needs of the facility. Therapy schedules are established similarly, so a therapy session at 2:00 p.m. may focus on dressing.

A session scheduled on Monday may focus on dressing; the Tuesday session may address bathing or toileting. In the home, these activities are part of a complete routine, the timing and sequence of which have been based on the needs and preferences of the patient and others living in the home. Moreover, that routine and many others are likely to be long established, automatic, and embedded in the specific locations in the home where they have been performed habitually. For most humans, habits and routines are not easily altered, especially those that are

---

1. This is a key difference between the *Outcome and Assessment Information Set* (OASIS) and other rating scales. The OASIS scores only selected aspects of activities of daily living and instrumental activities of daily living, but the score is based on performance in the home environment. This difference also explains why a patient may have scored higher on inpatient discharge assessment than on a corresponding OASIS item at the start of home health. OASIS scores are based on performance, not capacity. See Chapter 4 for more on the OASIS and documenting performance.

long-standing, even when the skills required to execute the specific actions have been lost or impaired. The presence of environmental cues—people, events, specific places in the home—reinforce habitual performance. This helps to explain why patients often fail to generalize what they learn in clinical settings—skills and techniques—when they return to the home or why they have difficulty initiating and sustaining new techniques even when they are taught in the home.

Roles are also relevant to performance. Roles imply specific patterns and constellations of activities. The roles a patient inhabits may be elicited by interviewing and discerned through cues in the environment. A display of dozens of family photos suggests a proud grandparent; the rifle cabinet and the eight-point buck mounted on the wall suggest a hunter. Roles also give meaning to performance. Getting dressed to attend a grandchild's recital or to go deer hunting with a buddy has a different meaning than sitting on a mat table and donning pajamas or sweatpants at the behest of a practitioner.

Activity demands elaborate on analysis of the activity to be performed. Activity demands include required body structures, body functions, and actions but also include contextual considerations. These considerations include aspects of the physical environment (objects used and space demands), aspects of the social context (social demands), and the temporality of the activity (sequencing and timing). Consideration of activity demands is important for analyzing occupations but is also important to introduce and to integrate modified strategies or adapted devices into existing routines.

The PEO (Law et al., 1996) offers a thinking frame for practice in the home that also accommodates the constructs of the ICF and the *Framework*. The PEO posits that there is an ongoing *transaction* between the person, the environment, and the occupation. Occupational performance is the (continual) *outcome* of this transaction. Occupational therapy in the home is different from occupational therapy in a clinic setting; the PEO can also be used to help the patient understand what to expect from occupational therapy.

Initial Visit

The purpose of the initial occupational therapy visit is to determine whether the patient needs occupational therapy services. If the need is present, the visit also includes identifying the outcomes and goals of occupational therapy and formulating the intervention plan that will achieve those outcomes.

Even if there already is a referral for occupational therapy that states specific interventions and frequencies, federal regulations require that an occupational therapist evaluate the patient's need for occupational therapy and develop a plan that is appropriate to and consistent with the evaluation findings ("Acceptance of Patients, Plan of Care, and Medical Supervision," 2002). No other discipline may evaluate either the need for occupational therapy or the type and intensity of intervention necessary to address such need.

Evaluation includes development of an occupational profile and the analysis of occupational performance.[2] What does this look like in home health? In most cases, it means eliciting information through multiple and even simultaneous means, forming hypotheses, and probing and analyzing to test these hypotheses, all while interacting with the patient (and, possibly, family members or caregivers). Such a process may seem too complex or overwhelming, but having a thinking frame helps to keep the process purposeful and organized. Table 5.2 offers a suggested process for gathering information. The first column describes the clinical reasoning that underpins the process. The second column is a suggested script to inform the patient or to elicit specific information or performance.

The suggested process involves gathering, analyzing, and refining information about the patient, environment, and daily occupations the patient has to perform. It answers these basic questions: What story have I entered? What was day-to-day life like for this person before the need for home health care? What is it like now, and why? The process begins with the patient's self-assessment of how he or she actually performs and also provides the practitioner the opportunity to observe both spontaneous and prompted performance of selected activities.

At the conclusion of the steps described in Table 5.2, the practitioner may assess select performance skills or body functions that require

---

2. For some payers other than Medicare, occupational therapy can conduct the home health start of care visit on rehab-only (non-nursing) referrals. This discussion focuses solely on the occupational therapy evaluation. Some of the items assessed are also collected for the home health comprehensive assessment, including OASIS.

TABLE 5.2
A Process to Assess Person, Environment, and Task Aspects of Performance During the Initial Occupational Therapy Evaluation Visit

Clinical reasoning and decision making	Suggested script
Explain why you are making the visit. Clearly identify that you are an occupational therapist. Give a simple explanation of what occupational therapy is and what you will be doing today and why. Note person–environment–occupation.	Your physician has requested that I see how you are doing with everyday activities. I'm an occupational therapist. In home health, occupational therapy focuses on the everyday things you have to do at home. There might be some things you are having difficulty doing or things you've had to give up or are thinking of giving up because they are taking too much effort or are feeling too risky. It helps me to know about the things you are used to doing, what your typical day is like, the places in the house where you get things done, and what you've been doing to keep doing them. I look at doing things as a puzzle with three pieces: what has to be done, what the tools or places are for the job, and what your body and mind have to do. I try to see how those pieces fit together, and if there's a problem, I work with the three parts so they fit together better. [Give one or more examples.] Does that make sense?
Obtain a recent occupational and health history. Note the social environment and current assistance (and, possibly, current assistance needs).	So, today, it helps if we start by letting me know more about you and what's been going on lately that got you referred for home health. Tell me about what you were used to doing before [the hospitalization, referral, fall, etc.]. Who lives here with you? Does anyone help you to go places? Get groceries or run errands? Keep the house? Do laundry? Get your meals? Help with things that folks usually do alone, like getting a bath or getting dressed? How often do you get out? Do you need help to go out? Tell me about that.
Note preferences, routines, and experiences.	How long have you lived here? What kind of work did you used to do [do you do]? What do you like to do to pass the time? It helps me to see where you have to do things. Can you show me around?

(Table continues)

Clinical reasoning and decision making	Suggested script
Segue to assessing performance while gathering information about skills, the environment, and activities (occupations).	OK, let's start out by showing me where you sleep.
Ask to be shown key areas of the home.	
Observe spontaneous mobility, spontaneous use of assistive device, and any assistance provided by the caregiver. Provide assistance only if necessary for safety.	
Engage the patient in conversation while moving from room to room. Ask about items or displays that may relate to family, hobbies, work, and achievements.	Are these your grandchildren? Tell me about the people in these photos. Did you make this _____? Is that trophy [award] yours? I see you have a lot of _____. Are you a _____?
Throughout the tour of the home, observe what the patient uses for support (furniture, doorknobs, etc.) and whether the patient needs to stop to engage in conversation, has dyspnea, or shows signs of fatigue. Take note of where telephones and exit doors are located, and note the presence of cordless phones and emergency response devices (e.g., Lifeline, Health Watch). Also observe whether the patient opens doors, manages lighting, or waits for you or the caregiver (if present) to do these tasks.	

(Table continues)

Clinical reasoning and decision making	Suggested script
Also look for evidence of problems: broken towel racks, loose doorknobs, alternative or auxiliary heat sources, poor illumination, and so on.	
Once in the bedroom, observe bed transfer and mobility. Assist only if necessary for safety.	Do you have any difficulty getting in or out of bed, rolling in the bed, or getting on or off the bed? Can you show me?
Segue to continence and toileting. Most patients will recognize this as a question about night toileting. If the answer is anything but no, follow up. If the patient uses a bedside commode, urinal, or bedpan, ask a follow-up question. Is the response consistent with observed skills?	How often do you have to get up at night? Do you ever have trouble making it in time? I know that's frustrating. Have you tried to do anything about that? What? Are you able to empty it OK?
Segue to the bathroom.	Let's see the bathroom.
If the patient is using a wheelchair, he or she may not be using the bathroom. But note what the patient (and caregiver, if present) does spontaneously. If the patient is using a walker, observe what he or she does with the walker to access the bathroom. Follow up on these observations.	That seems tricky. That seems like a lot of effort. Does it feel risky?
Visually assess the bathroom. Is there evidence that the tub or shower is used (or used for storage)? Note whether there are assistive devices in the bathroom.	Have you been using the raised toilet seat [grab bar, bath seat, transfer bench] for long? Is that working OK for you? Any problems? Is anyone helping you? The toilet is usually the lowest seat in the house. Any trouble getting on or off?

(Table continues)

Clinical reasoning and decision making	Suggested script
If there is no equipment or if selected items are not present, note the technique and what the patient uses for assistance.	Can you show me? Do you prefer to take a shower, a bath, or a sponge bath? [Don't ask if the patient already volunteered this information earlier.]
If the shower or tub appears to be used for storage and not for bathing, note whether the patient's mobility and environment indicate it is reasonable. Ask for a demonstration. Provide assistance only if necessary for safety, but provide close supervision.	How long has it been since you've been able to do that? Can you show me how you get in the tub or shower?
Before leaving the bathroom, ask how the patient functions in the bathroom. Some patients may need to rest at this point. If so, return to the room where the visit started and ask about the following issues. If the patient can tolerate it, segue to medications.	[Male patient:] How are you doing with shaving? [If the patient has a beard, ask about grooming the beard.] [Female patient:] How are you managing with doing your hair and putting on makeup?
Follow the patient to where the medications are kept. If the patient can't go there or doesn't know where they are kept, redirect to the next prompt and follow up later with the caregiver. If the patient retrieves medications, select one medication and probe. Note any discrepancies between what the patient reports and the instructions on the bottle.	Do you manage all of your medications by yourself, or does someone help you? Can you show me where they are? Where do you keep your medications? What is this medication for? When do you take it? Can you open the bottle, take a dose out, and close it up?

(Table continues)

Clinical reasoning and decision making	Suggested script
Assess fine motor skills for medication administration; put the medication back for the patient.	
If the patient can tolerate it and the tour has not yet moved to the kitchen, ask about meals.	Can we go on to the kitchen?
If the patient cannot access the kitchen, return to the room where the visit started and get a verbal report.	Do you fix any of your meals? Who gets your meals for you?
On the basis of the information the patient and caregiver have already provided, ask how meals are provided. If meals are being prepared by others, ask if the patient can get any snacks or drinks him- or herself.	If you were hungry or thirsty, could you get yourself a snack or a drink? Can you show me how you would get a drink or snack from the refrigerator? How would you carry it to the table [or the other room if there is no place to sit in the kitchen]? Let's return to the other room.
If retrieval is successful, redirect to where the visit started.	
While returning, note if a door is accessible to the patient or if he or she has to be wheeled or assisted. Would the patient be able to exit in an emergency, even with injuries?	What door is best for you to get in and out of the house? What would you do if you needed to get help in a hurry?
When everyone is again seated, segue to a safety response.	What if it were an emergency, like you smelled smoke?

(Table continues)

Clinical reasoning and decision making	Suggested script
If the initial response is to call family or a neighbor, ask what the number is (it may be programmed into phone; if so, the patient should be able to tell you how to access the programmed number).	
The only acceptable answers are 911 or the use of an emergency response unit and the patient is wearing the activator. If the patient does not offer an appropriate response, instruct him or her about 911 or the importance of wearing the activator.	
Segue to falls. Note the response and whether the patient hedges on falls (e.g., describes an incident as "not really a fall").	What would you do if you had a fall? Have you ever had a fall? When? Any others in the past few weeks or months? Were you hurt? What happened? Have you tried to do things to prevent having falls? What are they?
What is the patient's level of awareness and caution regarding the risk of falling?	
Conclude this part of the visit by returning to the patient's (and caregiver's) concerns.	Are there are other things you thought of while you were showing me around that you want me to know about?
Throughout the tour, you have been looking for cues and performance that either corroborate or contradict what the patient and caregiver reported at the start of the visit. This is a good point to stop and take a few minutes to organize the data you have gathered.	I need to sort through all that you've just told me about and showed me. I'm going to take a few minutes to make some notes and organize my thoughts before we proceed, OK?

more specific assessment. This approach saves time, as the patient's performance needs and priorities drive the selection of assessment rather than the practitioner's devoting time and effort assessing body functions or skills that are not related to performance priorities or concerns.

At this point, the practitioner evaluates the information gathered: the patient's concerns and priorities, the reported and observed performance, and the way the person–environment–occupation interaction supports or inhibits performance and data related to performance skills and body systems. Level of assistance is considered, as well as risk, effort, and the patient's satisfaction with performance.

The next question to be answered is, Where is this story going? The practitioner considers the patient's existing diagnoses and conditions and the patient's history and performance to evaluate the trajectory of the patient's current function. The patient may be on a *stable* trajectory, meaning that performance is consistent and predictable. The patient may be on an *ascending* trajectory, meaning that performance is improving and is likely to involve less assistance or effort or risk in the future. The patient may be on a *declining* trajectory, meaning that performance is deteriorating and that performance in the foreseeable future is expected to require more assistance or effort or involve more risk than it did today.

At this point, the practitioner needs to consider whether the existing trajectory is consistent with the occupational expectations and priorities of the patient (and caregiver) and whether occupational therapy is needed to achieve those expectations (and whether the expectations are consistent with the constraints of home health care). If the patient is on a declining trajectory, the question becomes, Will occupational therapy intervention be helpful to stabilize deteriorating performance?

If it appears the patient would benefit from occupational therapy, the next step is to identify what the outcomes of therapy might be. To accomplish this step, the practitioner should answer the question, If this patient receives occupational therapy, what will he or she look like when occupational therapy discharges? When the practitioner can answer these questions, the next step is to summarize the answers for the patient. Table 5.3 lists a framework for summarizing evaluation findings.

After sharing this information, the practitioner should allow the patient to confirm, elaborate on, or seek clarification on what the practitioner summarized. If the patient disagrees, the practitioner should ask

TABLE 5.3
Framework for Summarizing Evaluation Findings

Summary stem	Kinds of findings to include
These are things you told me are important to you.	Key patient priorities and concerns, Caregiver priorities and concerns, Baseline performance, Any report of falls or injuries, and Brief summary of daily routines or activity preferences.
These are the key things related to what you told me that are problems for you.	Focus first on strengths—effective strategies the patient uses and environmental features that support performance. Note effective assistance or cues used by the caregiver. Then focus on the activities the patient prioritized, and briefly summarize your analysis of each. Identify (analysis) the task, environment, or person factors that are problematic and/or can be addressed to yield improved performance or reduce risk or effort.
These are some things you didn't mention but I'm concerned about based on what you told me and what I observed.	Problems that the patient or caregiver seems to be unaware of or seems to disregard—this includes problems or potential problems for the caregiver, grossly unsafe techniques, fall hazards, fire hazards, and concerns about the patient being at home alone (emergency response, emergency egress, access to food and beverage, etc.); Dyspnea, if not acknowledged by the patient; Burden or risk to the caregiver; and Problems with medication management.

the patient to clarify and help the practitioner to make sense of what was observed or reported. The goal is a *shared understanding* of the patient's current situation, performance, and trajectory. From this shared understanding, the practitioner and patient together can refine the outcomes and goals initially projected by the practitioner. The practitioner may need to explain the transitional nature of home health and relate probable home health outcomes to longer term outcomes sought by the patient. The practitioner should also inform the patient of the projected frequency and duration of occupational therapy services and describe briefly the kinds of interventions anticipated.

Before leaving the home, the practitioner should clearly articulate several specific points to clarify expectations with the patient. Those points are listed in Table 5.4.

In cases where the patient lacks the cognitive ability to provide accurate or reliable information, the caregiver may be more actively involved in the interview and the tour of the house. However, the patient should be involved throughout the visit, including the establishment of goals and plans, to the extent he or she is willing and able to participate.

Intervention

With the goals identified with the patient and the plan to reach those goals formulated, the plan becomes the road map for intervention. This section describes key strategies and tools for intervention in home health. Intervention includes not only the services delivered *during* the home visit but also the aspects of practice that occur *between* visits.

The home visit is the most obvious aspect of home health practice. It is also the most resource intensive for both the agency and the practitioner. As a result, it is important to optimize the impact of each visit to move forward and achieve outcomes. Each visit should build on previous visits and lay a foundation for subsequent visits. Chapter 3 describes methods for evidence-based practice.

Communication is an important part of visits. It is important to communicate the purpose of any given intervention activity to the patient and caregivers, particularly because the everyday activities of occupational therapy can easily mask the therapeutic aspects. Distinguishing between occupation-based activities, purposeful activities, and preparatory methods is helpful when explaining to patients the difference between "building block functions or skills" (preparatory methods and some purposeful activities) and "actual doing" (occupation-based activities and some purposeful activities) (AOTA, 2002c). Occupation-

TABLE 5.4
Points to Clarify With the Patient
Prior to Concluding the Evaluation Visit

Key points	Why
Occupational therapy focuses on the patient's being able to perform the activities that he or she needs and wants to do. Performance depends on the fit between the person, the environment, and the task, so occupational therapy interventions address all three of these areas. This might be different from occupational therapy services the patient has received previously.	This avoids the perception that remediation of impairments is plan A and addressing the task or environment is plan B (or failure of plan A). It also avoids the perception that problems with performance are due to the patient's shortcomings.
Therapy is a collaboration. There are things the therapist and patient (and, in some cases, caregivers) will do together during therapy visits. There are also things that the patient will work on between visits, either alone or with the involvement of a caregiver. The things the patient does between visits are important because they help the patient to achieve the desired outcomes and to get the most from the therapy visits.	This discourages the expectation that progress is dependent on direct involvement of the therapist, strengthens the concept of a partnership, and also communicates to the patient and caregivers that caregiver participation is important.
There may be other things that can contribute to the outcomes that are not part of home health services or covered by insurers. If the therapist becomes aware of service or technology that would optimize desired goals, he or she will inform the patient and explain the pros and cons of the technology and how it might affect the outcomes that can be achieved. The decision as to whether to pursue the service or technology is solely the patient's.	This tempers the patient's expectations of home health services. It also makes it clear that the patient may need to invest resources in other services or technologies to optimize outcomes and that this decision resides with the patient, not the therapist or the agency.
The job of both the patient and the therapist is to put the therapist out of a job.	Discharge means success, not abandonment or failure.

based activity is focused not only on accomplishing the task but also on achieving a better match between what the patient can do and what the environment provides so that the patient is better equipped for performance at the next opportunity. The distinction between skill building and actual in-context performance is helpful to communicate to the patient and caregiver, to the team, and in documentation so that the focus of occupational therapy intervention and expertise is clearly articulated.

Many practitioners new to home care find themselves at a loss about what to do and what to use in the absence of the preparatory and purposeful activity tools typically found in clinics. Stacking cones, pegboards, pulleys, puzzles, and other equipment that are considered essential in many clinics become unnecessary in home care. Finding ways to open pill bottles, operate lamp switches, turn door locks, and open food containers provides the patient with plentiful, practical opportunities to challenge fine motor skills. Folding laundry, sorting clothing, organizing pantries, washing windows, and hanging clothes challenge balance and upper body strength in ways that are more functional than any clinic activity. Rather than seeking contrived activities that challenge only isolated skills, home care encourages the patient to actually perform the daily activities that are presenting challenges (occupation-based activities). Thus, occupation is a process and a product.

A patient at home cannot wait for deficits to resolve before engaging in daily occupations. A patient has to eat, regardless of how precise his or her grasp is on a utensil. A patient cannot wait to use the toilet until the transfer is perfect. Compensation must be addressed from the first visit, along with remediation if it is appropriate. An emphasis on remediating deficits without at least equal emphasis on facilitating actual performance (with or without compensation) will lead patients to believe that we can fix impairments that are not remediable. It also sets the stage for any later emphasis on compensation to be perceived as a second-best solution when remediation has failed.

To optimize the value of visits, patients and caregivers need to appreciate the importance of what occurs *between* visits. Both patients and practitioners have responsibilities between visits. Practitioner responsibilities include communication and coordination with other disciplines and, at times, the physician. Coordination may also include arranging for equipment or resources needed to progress the plan of care. Finally, the time between visits provides the practitioner an opportunity to monitor the patient by telephone.

Some patients will perceive therapy as something the practitioner does *to* the patient or think that home programs are activities the patient is supposed to do *for* the practitioner. Some patients may feel that progress can happen only if the practitioner is involved, discounting the power of their own adaptive responses and minimizing the role of the caregiver. Caregivers are integral to the therapy process; they are not merely an extra set of hands doing *for* the patient. For progress to occur, it is essential that patients have homework between visits. In many cases, homework includes the involvement of a caregiver. It is important to emphasize the partnership and instill ownership in the patient and the caregiver.

One approach is to explain to the patient that the activities addressed in occupational therapy fall into three categories. The first category includes activities that are done only when the practitioner is present. These activities are new or complicated or have significant risk involved and require that the practitioner be present and involved for them to be done safely.

As the patient progresses, the goal is to move activities into the second category. In this category the patient can do the activity well enough that the practitioner does not have to be present. However, someone else still has to be present and involved to cue, monitor, supervise, and/or complete the task if the patient is unable to complete it. This is where caregivers become important in giving the patient as many opportunities as possible to practice or carry out the activity in a safe, supervised manner. The caregiver *supervises* or *assists* in the activity rather than doing it. Once an activity moves into this category, it is not addressed during the visits unless the patient or caregiver identifies problems or it is time to reassess to see whether it should move to the third category.

The third category consists of activities that the patient can perform without a caregiver present but performance needs continued refinement (to reduce effort or time, to refine the result). These activities should be performed every time the patient gets an opportunity and should *not* be performed by caregivers. When performance requires the incorporation of new or adapted strategies, patients begin to generalize strategies to new situations and to identify and implement self-initiated adaptations.

One approach is to leave it up to the patient and caregiver to decide when activities move from the second category to the third. This emphasizes that their own ability to assess and appraise performance is more important than what the practitioner says. However, for some activities where disagreement exists or where risk is higher, the practitioner should be involved in determining when performance progresses to the third category. The two most common activities that fit this description are bathing and cooking. Because these involve significant risk, the practitioner may prefer to directly assess performance before recommending that the patient perform the activity without supervision. Once the practitioner has the opportunity to reassess, the patient, caregiver, and practitioner can decide whether the patient is ready to go solo.

Phone calls to the patient between visits offer a means to encourage and monitor activities that have moved to the second and third categories. Checking in with the patient between visits maintains continuity from visit to visit, reinforces the importance of homework, and offers an opportunity to problem solve if the patient or caregiver is encountering difficulty implementing homework. In some cases, a phone call may result in a change in the expected visit schedule.

Homework is not the same thing as a home program. The latter term typically refers to exercises or care and management of an orthotics or similar device. A home program may be one aspect of homework, but there are many other activities that fall in this domain. All activities in the second and third categories are homework. Some kinds of homework pertain to the environment. These include making environmental changes to facilitate performance (e.g., rearranging furniture) and obtaining tools or equipment (e.g., purchasing a bath seat). Homework pertaining to the environment typically requires the involvement of a caregiver, as do activities in the second category.

Self-care activities that fit in the second category are appropriate to delegate to a home health aide if no willing caregiver is available. The patient's need for only supervised repetitive practice to improve skills is not a justification for skilled occupational therapy, and these activities should not be occurring during occupational therapy visits. Delegating the repetitive practice to aides or caregivers allows precious therapy time to be focused on tasks that do require the skills of a practitioner. In all cases where aides are involved, the occupational therapist should ensure that the aide care plan is coordinated with the patient's progress in ADL and that the assistance provided by the aide is consistent with the patient's emerging performance.

Contextual Intervention: Physical Barriers and Safety Issues

Because most homes in this country have not been designed with accessibility in mind, practice in the home includes dealing with problems that do not arise in other settings. Accessibility issues are most obvious when a patient is using a wheelchair, but ambulatory individuals may also face significant challenges in the home. Potential challenges include stairs, uneven flooring, thick pile carpet, heavy doors, furniture obstacles, clutter, pets, and narrow passages and doorways that do not accommodate walkers. Bathroom doorways are usually the narrowest in the home. In the bathroom the toilet seat is typically low, and the side of the tub or shower is high. There is seldom a grab bar, but there are many handy substitutes, such as faucets, doorknobs, soap dishes, towel racks, and the edge of the sink. These substitutes are not designed to provide support, but patients may have depended on them for stabilization or support well before they were referred to home health care. These devices are never safe to use in this manner, but patients may be convinced of their utility and deny the risk.

Sometimes home delivery of durable medical equipment has been arranged when patients leave a rehabilitation facility. This often means the home health care practitioner arrives in time to discover that the standard adult wheelchair is too wide to make the turn from a hallway to the bedroom or that the bath seat is incompatible with the configuration of the tub or shower. A portion of the first home visit may be spent arranging pickup of inappropriate durable medical equipment and ordering devices that are immediately necessary.

Design features also create more subtle challenges. Thermostats may be inaccessible, and phone jacks may be located in rooms that the patient cannot access. Lighting controls, whether wall mounted or on a lamp fixture, may be inaccessible as well. The entry doors may be difficult for the patient to reach, which creates a risk in terms of emergency egress. This may also present a logistical challenge for you: The patient may have difficulty getting to the door to admit you, and the alternative, leaving the door unlocked, presents a personal safety risk. There may be no counters or tables near stoves, microwave ovens, and refrigerators where the patient can place hot or heavy items once they are retrieved from the appliances. A heavy refrigerator door may be a barrier and may swing with enough force to knock the patient off balance.

As mentioned previously, *risk* is an essential issue to address in home care. In the home the physical environment may complicate performance by posing challenges that compromise safety. There may be aspects of the environment that are inherently unsafe, such as fire hazards or conditions that limit personal security. However, most other aspects of the environment do not pose an inherent risk. Instead, the risk must be assessed based on the interaction of the person and the environment.

Many home health patients live alone or are home alone without assistance for a significant portion of the day. Just because a patient or caregiver states that a task is performed without assistance does not mean it can be considered independent, which implies safe performance. It is essential to consider safety as an essential element of performance. From a practical perspective, it is not within the power of the practitioner or the patient to ensure safety. However, it is possible for the practitioner and the patient to work together to reduce risk associated with performance.

Some safety concerns are exclusively a function of the environment, and altering the environment will reduce the risk factor. Other safety concerns are a function of the interaction of the person, environment, and task. What does this mean? During the past decade, many organizations, from home improvement stores to insurance companies, have developed home safety checklists. These lists are used to screen for the presence or absence of specific conditions or features in the home, with instruction on how the condition or feature should be modified to improve safety. What these checklists fail to consider is that risk is introduced when habitual performance is disrupted by alterations in a familiar environment where performance is embedded. Especially for an older adult who has lived in a dwelling for many years, changing the environment solely on the basis of a checklist, without taking into account actual, habitual, spontaneous performance, can effectively increase, rather than decrease, the risk or uncertainty associated with daily activities.

For practitioners who wish to use a safety assessment that is designed for the home environment and oriented to performance, the *SAFER-HOME (Safety Assessment of Function and the Environment for*

Rehabilitation-Health Outcome Measurement and Evaluation) is an oc-cupational therapy health outcomes assessment developed by commu-nity-based practitioners in Canada for use with patients in their homes (Community Occupational Therapists and Associates Health, 2006).

Many patients and their caregivers resist efforts to address risk sim-ply because they "don't want to think about what could happen." It is important to discuss safety issues in as nonthreatening a manner as pos-sible and to ensure that the patient and significant caregivers are aware of risks and how they can be minimized. Home health agencies are mandated to assess safety and risk. The discussion and recommendations should also be documented. In the event that a patient sustains an injury, both you and your agency will want the patient record to show clearly that you made the patient aware of risks and the patient's response to such information. Patients and their caregivers may choose to disregard such information, but it is incumbent on the practitioner to make them aware of risks and to recommend strategies to reduce the risk.

Some patients may feel uneasy about being left alone in the home but have not raised the issue with caregivers because they don't want to add to the caregiving burden and are aware that the person needs to leave. Articulating the risks and identifying potential solutions may help the patient to acknowledge these concerns and recognize that there are reasonable means to reduce risk. Simply having a cordless phone nearby may ease a patient's anxiety and reduce the burden on caregivers.

Reducing risk is not the only reason for assessing spontaneous per-formance in the home environment. Many daily occupations are *em-bedded* in the environment. This means that performance is not simply a product of the person–environment–occupation interaction; perfor-mance is facilitated by the environment. For many long-established occupations, cues in the environment prompt performance without requiring the conscious attention of the person. When performance is disrupted by injury or illness, the fit between the person, the environ-ment, and the task may also be disrupted. Modifying the environment to reduce demands may reestablish the fit and reestablish effective and satisfying performance.

Environmental modifications fall in three broad categories: (a) in-troduction of tools and devices, (b) reconfiguration of materials in the existing environment, and (c) alteration of architectural features. Assis-tive tools and devices are also common in other practice settings. How-ever, routine occupations in the home may require tools or devices, in addition to items such as bath seats, reachers, and shoehorns, that are not common and may even be completely customized for the patient. For example, management of the environment (ventilation, illumination, security) is an instrumental activity of daily living that might require tools or devices to manage tasks such as locking and unlocking doors or turning on lights. Reconfiguration is an environmental intervention strategy that is often used by practitioners but is seldom identified as such. Reconfiguration refers to rearranging objects in the environment to achieve a better fit among the person, environment, and occupation. Common examples of reconfiguration include reorganizing the contents of a pantry or cupboard to reduce bending, reaching, or putting excessive stress on joints or rearranging the furniture in a room to optimize access for a walker or wheelchair. Alteration of structural and architectural features refers to construction, remodeling, and alteration of permanent features of the home. Examples include constructing ramps, installing curbless showers, increasing the width of doorways, and installing higher toilet fixtures.

Medicare and most health care insurers do not cover most assistive devices and do not cover structural alterations. However, environmental modifications can make a significant difference in the person–environment–occupation dynamic and, thus, performance. Sometimes home health practitioners are reluctant to mention environmental modifications because of the lack of insurance coverage. However, it is important for patients and caregivers to make *informed choices* about options that may enhance performance. The practitioner can also provide important information about how a proposed modification can affect performance, in relation not only to home care outcomes but also to the patient's and caregiver's longer term performance.

For example, a patient is currently sponge bathing while seated at bedside, with assistance provided to set up the task and to wash lower legs and feet. The practitioner has assessed performance in terms of the patient's abilities, the demands of the tasks, and the environment. In the practitioner's clinical judgment, the introduction of a bath seat, handheld shower, and long-handled bath brush would offer a better fit for the patient's skills and enable the patient to perform a seated shower. With practice, the practitioner expects that the patient would be able to perform the seated shower without assistance or setup. Without these environmental modifications, the practitioner estimates that the patient's skills will improve only to the point where sponge bathing could be performed while seated at the sink, or showering would have to be assisted to manage effort and risk. The practitioner informs the patient and caregiver of these two projected outcomes and also provides information about approximate costs of the recommended devices. This approach allows the patient (or patient and caregiver) to understand the impact of purchasing (or not purchasing) the items on outcomes of occupational therapy, to select the preferred outcome, and to then purchase (or decline to purchase) the items. If the patient opts to purchase equipment, the practitioner may then provide information about vendors or suppliers so the patient can select a vendor and purchase the items.

As mentioned earlier, sometimes practitioners are reluctant to address equipment because of the lack of third-party coverage and potential costs to the patient. Making equipment recommendations in relation to outcomes enables the patient and caregiver to evaluate purchases in terms of *all* costs, not solely in dollars. For the patient, having to give up showers or to secure assistance to the shower may be a greater cost than the expense of the equipment. For the caregiver, having to be present to assist with the shower on a regular basis may cost time away from work or family. And if hired assistance is considered, the ongoing cost may be considerably higher than the onetime cost of the equipment. Without the information about equipment *and* outcomes, a patient may decline equipment, believing that occupational therapy will result in improvement of skills adequate to shower independently. This may result in unrealized expectations and disappointment with occupational therapy. For the practitioner, explicitly linking proposed interventions to outcomes enables the patient to make informed choices and promotes shared outcome expectations.

Contextual Intervention: Working With Caregivers

One of the unique features of home health care is the involvement of family and friends in the coordination of care. Unlike settings that employ aides, technicians, or other paraprofessionals, home care relies largely on the services of unpaid, inexperienced caregivers. Indeed, one of the functions of home health intervention is to equip these caregivers with the skills to take over responsibility for ongoing care as professional services are phased out.

The difference between these caregivers and paraprofessionals cannot be overstated. Whereas paraprofessionals are paid for work they have chosen to do, volunteer caregivers are usually involved because of their relationship or proximity to the patient. Their role as caregiver may be as new and accidental as the patient's illness or disease. Moreover, paraprofessionals do their job day in and day out, with a variety of patients or clients, but caregivers are usually new to the job and work with only one patient.

In addition, the caregiver has an emotional tie to the patient and an emotional and sometimes financial stake in the outcomes of care. A willing, invested caregiver can make a strong contribution to outcomes, but it is a mistake to assume that, because a caregiver is present, he or she is willing and invested.

Any accident or illness that results in a need for home care is likely to result in an alteration in roles and role performance. This alteration affects family and friends as well as the patient. A breadwinner may become a dependent. A daughter may find herself changing her father's diapers. A son may have to learn to dose insulin syringes for his mother. And a spouse who has never managed the finances, cooked a meal, had the car repaired, or done the laundry may suddenly be thrust into new responsibilities *in addition* to the role of caregiver. In some cases a grown child may find himself or herself in the "parent" role with Mother or Father, a role reversal that the patient may resent and resist.

Grudges and grievances that have been dormant for years may suddenly flare up in a health crisis. A daughter who resents her father for divorcing her mother may act out that resentment when called on to be the father's caregiver. A spouse who has felt neglected may become excessively dependent and demanding of the partner who is now obligated to provide care. When siblings (and their spouses) are called on to work together to care for a parent, long-standing rivalries can ignite. The caregiver and patient may have a positive, affirming relationship, or they may have a dysfunctional relationship that has persisted for years.

Caregivers may be willing volunteers or unwilling conscripts. A few have prior experience as caregivers, but most have no experience at all. Even a nurse or practitioner with years of experience will be thrust into a new role when called on to be a caregiver to a spouse, parent, or sibling. Whatever the dynamic, family caregivers wield the greatest influence for success or for sabotage of our therapeutic interventions. The best therapy in the world will not be effective if the key caregivers do not support it.

What does this mean for you? Most simply it means ignore care-givers at your peril. Never assume that therapy involves just the patient and you. Rarely will a patient in home care have no significant others involved in care; the intensity of care needs implied by homebound status usually necessitates assistance from others.

The *social context* of caregivers, friends, and family members around the patient will influence interventions. This means that assessing and addressing the social context is an essential aspect of a deliberate, client-centered approach to home care. The abilities, limitations, and expectations of the social context are just as significant as the affordances and barriers encountered in the physical context. The behaviors of caregivers and their interactions with the patient also provide additional clues to the *cultural context*. Values and beliefs regarding the role of a person who is ill or disabled, and the obligations of the family, are culturally based, and they vary widely in our society. What outside professionals may perceive as fostering dependence may actually be a culturally based imperative to show honor and care for a respected elder. Apparent ambivalence on the part of a caregiver may actually be deference to the patient's autonomy and self-determination. A family with a strong work ethic may have difficulty appreciating interventions that are designed to conserve energy and simplify tasks, and the patient who tries to implement these strategies may be misconstrued as lazy or may even perceive himself or herself as giving in by using such techniques. Time and effort spent to clarify expectations and verify inferences will contribute to outcomes that are meaningful and sustainable.

There are two additional areas where nonprofessional caregivers are very different from paraprofessionals and where you must interact with them differently. First, it is easy to forget that they have their own lives. Whereas paraprofessionals are paid for the job of caring for others, caregivers are usually providing care *in addition to* their other roles and daily responsibilities. You need to seek cues from caregivers to avoid overburdening them. You need to express an understanding that they have other responsibilities, and you need to credit them for their contribution to home care. A sensitive approach will build alliances that foster caregiver cooperation and optimize the effectiveness of interventions.

The second area is underestimating the gap in knowledge and expertise between trained professionals and the volunteer caregivers we instruct. Paraprofessionals soon become familiar with facility protocols and professional jargon, but caregivers are new to this business of therapy. It is your professional responsibility to bridge the gap between your expertise and the patient's and caregiver's knowledge so that you can give instructions and recommendations at a level that is meaningful to them. This includes consideration of their ability to assimilate new learning and the difficulty of altering lifelong habits. Instruction may need to be provided in alternative formats if poor literacy, low English proficiency, or visual impairments limit the effectiveness of written instruction.

To teach patients and caregivers effectively, you may also need to spend time explaining not only *what* you want them to do but *why*. The rationale may be obvious to you, but you should never assume that it is obvious to the patient or the caregiver. In the example mentioned previously, teaching energy conservation may seem counterproductive to a caregiver who is convinced that the patient is weak and just has to exercise to get stronger. The caregiver is unlikely to appreciate that simply participating in self-care or eating a meal is fatiguing for the patient. Explaining the reasons for energy conservation enables the patient and the caregiver to make informed choices about implementing such instruction.

At times a caregiver will report that a patient will perform activities for the practitioner but not for the caregiver. In some instances this situation is rooted in the relationship between the caregiver and the patient. Whenever this is reported, it may be a sign of a gap between the assistance and cues provided by the practitioner, which are enabling performance, and the assistance and cues provided by the caregiver, which are inadequate to support the same level of performance. Reflect on this possibility and if possible directly assess the patient's performance with the caregiver providing the assistance. In many instances simple verbal cues or environmental adjustments that practitioners make without thinking about them are the keys to enabling successful performance. It is your responsibility to make that tacit knowledge plain and understandable to the caregiver. It is easy to focus on the physical assistance you want the caregiver to provide and forget to explain the environmental setup and verbal cues.

Explaining the *why* is also essential whenever we want a caregiver to do something that seems to take more time or effort than the method that seems obvious to the person. For example, a caregiver may find it simpler to pull a patient up from the bed to a sitting position rather than take the time to allow the patient to roll to the side while lying and then make the transition to sitting on the side of the bed, especially if this is difficult for the patient. The explanation should include the importance of the caregiver's protecting his or her back while helping the patient. The caregiver should also understand that the patient's additional effort yields improvements in strength, confidence, and control of movement. Such explanation avoids terms such as *joint protection, motor learning, transfers, weight shift,* and other jargon that may confuse the caregiver.

Outcomes

Working on reestablishing a daily routine directed by the patient (rather than the schedule of home health visits) is essential for health maintenance such as medication scheduling and adequate nutrition. It is also essential to maintain orientation and memory. Identifying valued activities and ways to accomplish them gives the patient a reason to get up and get going in the morning, as well as an opportunity to rediscover skills and knowledge. If you emphasize performance of specific tasks (bathing, dressing, preparing meals) without identifying how these will fit together into a workable routine, we leave a large task for the patient to tackle after we are gone. In recent years, Medicare has put an increasing emphasis on outcomes, specifically outcomes that help to sustain the patient in the home. Occupational therapy intervention, which reestablishes routines and supports roles and habits, provides the framework to *sustain* performance after therapy, and home care, are discontinued. In many cases, patients continue an *improvement trajectory* after discharge, as they generalize strategies, refine performance, and engage in an expanding repertoire of occupations.

When patients, caregivers, and practitioners agree on desired outcomes at the start of home care, discharge becomes a graduation from therapy rather than a termination. Discharge does not mean that no further improvement in performance is possible, only that improving or sustaining performance no longer requires the involvement of the practitioner. If discharge occurs because a patient is no longer homebound, then discharge also may be a transition to therapy that addresses still broader skills (community reentry) on an outpatient basis. This approach makes it clear to patients that their job is to put you out of a job.

Home care practitioners of all disciplines sometimes complain that they have little control over what patients or caregivers do and that this lack of control inhibits them from accomplishing their care goals. *Noncompliance* is a term that is often used to refer to patient behavior that is inconsistent with the instructions and expectations of the practitioner. In home care the noncompliant label takes on questionable validity and relevance. *Compliance* implies a hierarchical relationship where *obedience* is expected. This view of the practitioner–client relationship is inconsistent with the values of occupational therapy, which emphasize collaboration and a client-centered approach. In recent years, a growing number of quality and standard-setting bodies in health care have recommended a shift away from a practitioner-centered, compliance-oriented approach to a client-centered (or patient-centered) approach that recognizes and respects the patient as the "source of control" (Institute of Medicine, 2001, p. 61). Expecting compliance in a setting where they have so little control is likely to lead to frustrated practitioners whom patients and caregivers perceive as bossy and demanding.

Patient self-management is an increasingly important outcome in health care. Explained simply, self-management is the ability to effectively manage one's own health and daily activities to one's own satisfaction. Self-management support is the process of making changes in health care and the community to facilitate patient self-management (Glasgow, Davis, Funnell, & Beck, 2003). Applied to home care, the role of the practitioners is self-management, and the outcome is self-management. From this perspective, the expectation of intervention is not patient compliance but patient confidence in his or her own ability as a self-manager (Quality Insights of Pennsylvania, 2007). In contrast to approaches that emphasize patient education, where the patient parrots back information or demonstrates isolated skills, self-management emphasizes patient behavior and routines.

The growing emphasis on patient self-management has several implications for occupational therapy practice in home health. Recognition and respect for client control is consistent with the history and values of occupational therapy. The emphasis on patient behavior—doing—relates directly to occupations. This includes both occupations directly related to health, such as administering medications, and occupations that involve overall care for oneself (ADL). Self-management also relates to performance patterns—the establishment or reestablishment of habits and routines that incorporate and integrate health management into routines of daily living.

There is an additional implication that is also a significant departure from occupational therapy in most other health care settings. Self-management is a desirable outcome regardless of diagnosis. In fact, patient self-management emerged as an approach to dealing with chronic illnesses. Many of the patients referred for home health care have one or more chronic conditions, the most common of which are heart failure and diabetes. These are often the most complex and challenging patients, yet because these conditions are not associated with rehab, these patients are seldom referred for occupational therapy. However, occupational therapy intervention can be powerful self-management support that is focused on the performance of self-management activities and the establishment of self-management routines. As agencies face the growing challenge of providing self-management support for patients with chronic conditions, home health offers occupational therapy practitioners an opportunity. Although conditions such as diabetes and heart failure may not be as familiar as stroke and arthritis, individuals living with these conditions may benefit from occupational therapy to incorporate health management into daily routines.

Home Care From the Patient's Perspective

One facet of home care that is not discussed often enough is the experience of homebound patients. It is difficult to imagine what it is like to be a prisoner in your own home, betrayed by your own body or mind and further restricted by barriers in the home that had never been barriers before. The place where you feel most in control and that most reflects your life, your values, and your personality becomes a place that mocks your sense of self and holds you captive. The simple acts of entering and exiting the house, going to your car and driving away, or stopping for a bite to eat or to pick up a loaf of bread are all luxuries that are out of reach of the patients you treat every day. It is important to recognize the psychological effect of being homebound and of being held captive by one's own home. The simple activities that you take for granted every day present challenges or sometimes insurmountable obstacles to your patients.

It is important for your patients to know that you appreciate what they are experiencing, even if you cannot really understand it. Few practitioners have had the experience of being homebound because of illness or injury, especially if the illness is chronic or the injury results in permanent losses of body structures or body functions. Even fewer practitioners have had the experience of being unable to perform taken-for-granted daily activities or of needing assistance to accomplish activities that have been performed with little thought or effort since childhood.

Regardless of how many homebound patients you encounter, every patient's situation is unique, as is that patient's story. The effort to appreciate circumstances from the patient's perspective fosters empathy. That empathy is the foundation of a trusting, collaborative relationship. The ordinary "doing" of a therapy session takes on multiple meanings, as both a means to an end (outcomes) and as an end itself as the patient has an opportunity to reengage in activities that hold purpose and meaning (Clark, 1993). This is especially important when current performance challenges seem far removed from previous or hoped-for achievements. Even routine activities such as dressing may have meanings associated with the past (the favorite sweater that was a gift from a friend), present (being able to don street clothes instead of pajamas and a robe), and future (the expectation of dressing up to attend an upcoming family celebration). For a brief period, the practitioner and the therapy become part of the larger story—the patient's story.

Case Example: Tommy's Story

Tommy was a man in his late 20s who sustained severe injuries in a motorcycle accident. He had multiple fractures of scapula, ribs, vertebrae, and bones in one leg. He destroyed his knee joint and lost most of the skin on the leg. He had a compression injury to the spinal cord. He was discharged from rehab to home health with his leg in an immobilizer (with dressing in place over extensive grafts), a TLSO (thoracic-lumbar-sacral orthosis) brace that had to be worn at all times except in supine, and a self-catheterization and bowel regimen. During the initial evaluation I found out that he was a computer engineer who had moved up to management in his company, that he was a high school soccer star who still played in a league, and that he lived in a nearby city but had been discharged to the rural home of his parents, who were his primary caregivers. He was their only son.

During the initial visit, the physical therapist was also present. With effort and assistance, Tommy got his brace on, got up onto the side of the bed, and walked with crutches about 20 feet. He was exhausted by the time he got back to the bed, and it took several more minutes and maneuvers to remove the brace and get him positioned in bed. The physical therapist announced that the goal she had decided on was for Tommy to get to the back door and back to his room by himself on his crutches. The physical therapist told him she'd "leave the uppers" to me, because we "split you in the middle." Unable to let that comment go by without a response, I announced, "That's good, at least I get to work with your brain."

Tommy was desperate to get to the point where there was not a relative sitting by his side all day. He was also bored. I told him that I would work with him to figure out how he could manage so his mother could go back to work and to see if we could find some activities that would stave off boredom.

Tommy and I worked on getting his brace on, getting off the bed, and transferring to his wheelchair. We found a way for him to carry his reacher and his cordless phone on his wheelchair, and we got a lap desk that would hold his laptop computer. I located an Internet provider with a local phone access number (rare in his rural area), and Tommy logged on to his Web page to show me photos of his other motorcycle (which was now for sale) and his family and to tell me about his job. He talked about traveling and how he loved sports. He made plans to get his mother back to work.

We worked out the logistics for Tommy to get to the kitchen in his wheelchair and fix himself a sandwich. The first attempt took more than an hour from the bed to the finished sandwich, but he knew he could do it. Once his family understood how things had to be arranged in the refrigerator so he could reach them, we knew he could fix his own lunch. Assuring his mother that the cordless phone would always be within reach, he persuaded her to go back to work. That first day back, she called to check on him every 15 minutes, but he had accomplished his first big goal: to be able to stay alone in the house. In the meantime the physical therapist was working with Tommy on getting in and out of the house and down the steps with his crutches.

When the skin grafts had healed adequately, his doctor allowed him to shower. We figured out the transfer and arranged for a bath seat, and Tommy drained the hot water tank when he took his first shower in 3 months. Tommy started coming up with adaptations and techniques on his own, or he would call me with a problem and a potential solution to get my feedback or ideas to make it even better. Our next challenge was getting him back to his own (multilevel) home.

We arranged for a family member to transport him to his town-house, and I met him there. A narrow flight of stairs, with thick carpet and angled steps at a turn, was a huge challenge. We assessed the rest of the house, he made notes about modifications that I recommended, and we decided that it was best that he stay with his parents until he was more mobile.

That was the last visit I had with Tommy. After a few more phone calls, we decided he had put me out of a job, and he was starting to get vocational rehabilitation as he made plans to go back to work. He phoned me when he moved back to his townhouse, and he told me he was arranging for his 6-year-old daughter, who had been living with him before the accident, to come back to live with him. He was excited that he could be a dad again.

A week before that last visit, I had an OT student with me for Level I fieldwork. She asked him how he thought he was doing in therapy. He asked, "OT-wise or PT-wise?" She asked him what he thought the difference was. He said, "Well, the physical therapists are working on getting me stronger, getting me up and moving. But OT, you guys are helping me get my life back." Tommy got his life back, and we had the privilege of contributing to the work he did to make a new life after his accident.

Conclusion

The day-to-day practice of home care is challenging, rewarding, and never dull. It is incredibly rich and complex and demands that you use clinical reasoning skills constantly and be able to think on your feet. Home care practice offers you the incredible privilege of stepping into the life space and life story of a patient and family to create a new or revised story. Occupational therapy is uniquely prepared to respond to recent and emerging home health care initiatives that emphasize functional, sustainable outcomes and self-management. Practice is holistic and patient centered, with unique opportunities to assess and address the person, environment, and occupation to facilitate performance that is meaningful to the patient. It allows you to address very practical problems (How will Mrs. Smith bathe?) with creativity (Do we change the environment, alter the task, or do something else entirely?) and collaborate with the patient to produce meaningful outcomes. Home health brings together the art and science of practice in a setting that grounds you in the practical realities of occupation. And for those practitioners who have worked in home care, the home is the only clinic they will ever need.

Fieldwork Education in Home Health

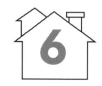

6

Carol Siebert, MS, OTR/L, FAOTA

Fieldwork in home health presents opportunities for students, practitioners, occupational therapy educational programs, and home health agencies. Students have the opportunity to experience practice in a natural environment—the home. Practitioners have the opportunity to share their expertise and expand their professional roles. Academic fieldwork coordinators have the opportunity to expand their roster of fieldwork sites and establish successful collaborations with home health agencies. Agencies have the opportunity to expand the population of practitioners interested in and prepared for home health practice.

Establishing a fieldwork site requires a commitment on the part of the agency, the educational program, and the practitioners who will serve as clinical educators. This chapter addresses the issues that fieldwork coordinators, practitioners, and home health agencies must address to create a successful clinical fieldwork collaboration. This chapter contains four stand-alone sections. The first section is directed to academic fieldwork coordinators to acquaint them with home health practice, including factors that must be considered when assigning students to home health fieldwork. The second section is directed to home health occupational therapy practitioners to acquaint them with the responsibilities and preparatory tasks associated with establishing a home health fieldwork site. The third section is directed to home health agency administrators and managers to acquaint them with the requirements and responsibilities associated with establishing a home health fieldwork site. The final section summarizes key principles for all three groups to establish a successful occupational therapy *fieldwork experience*.

Academic Fieldwork Coordinators: What You Need to Know About Home Health

Fieldwork in home health is an opportunity for students to be exposed to practice in a client's natural environment. This makes home health an attractive fieldwork option for both students and academic fieldwork coordinators. However, although home health fieldwork may be perceived as a "community" practice setting, home health is a highly regulated setting that is strongly influenced by payer coverage criteria. Home health is also regulated at state and federal levels, with regulations based on medical models of service delivery. Home health is a community practice setting in the sense that practice occurs within the community instead of in a facility, but in all other respects, home health is medical model practice.

Many educational programs categorize fieldwork sites according to the primary population served and the type of problems that precipitate occupational therapy referrals. Home health is not easily categorized. Because Medicare is the dominant influence in home health practice, most clients served by home health are older adults or adults who have a permanent disability that qualifies them for Medicare benefits. Although young adults and sometimes children are served by home health agencies, these referrals typically compose less than 5% of all occupational therapy referrals in home health. A broad range of impairments or diagnoses are found among the client population in home health. These may include diagnoses common in rehabilitation settings, such as stroke, acquired brain injury, osteoarthritis, rheumatoid arthritis, and a variety of neurodegenerative conditions. Some home health agencies offer behavioral health programs, and occupational therapy may be included in those programs. In these cases, individuals with mood disorders or schizophrenia may also be represented in the occupational therapy caseload. Home health is also a part of postsurgical care, so clients who have undergone orthopedic repairs, joint replacements, and vascular surgeries with amputations may also be part of the occupational therapy caseload. It is also common for clients receiving home health care to have multiple chronic conditions, such as diabetes, chronic obstructive pulmonary disease, congestive heart failure, and acquired immune deficiency syndrome (AIDS). It is not uncommon for clients to be admitted to home health care following an acute exacerbation or complication of a chronic condition. With this wide variety of problems and conditions represented in the occupational therapy caseload, home health fieldwork can best be described as a generalist experience with an adult population, primarily older adults 60 years of age and older.

There are aspects of home health practice that may make it unsuitable for fieldwork for some students. Home health is sometimes seen as a flexible fieldwork option because the practitioners may not be on a rigid 8-to-5 schedule within a facility. However, most home health practitioners have a regular schedule for starting and ending the day and are on the road or conducting visits throughout the course of the day. Some practitioners stop for lunch, whereas others may not. Traffic, unexpected problems during a visit, or inclement weather may prolong the workday. Because home care practitioners are on the road, many bring their lunch or snacks and eat in the car. Even taking bathroom breaks depends on the availability of public restrooms or whether clients in the caseload permit the practitioner to use their bathroom. For all of these reasons, home health is not a good option for students who need a predictable schedule with predictable breaks, especially if those breaks are needed to rest, eat, or administer medication. It is also not a suitable fieldwork site for students who need to end the day at a specific time (e.g., to meet child care pickup times, etc.). Finally, home health is not viable placement option for students who have limited tolerance for traveling in a vehicle. During the 12-week Level II fieldwork, a student and practitioner may log as many as 5,000 miles in a vehicle. Even in a single week of Level I fieldwork, a student and practitioner may log as many as 500 miles. Students who have limited tolerance for car travel should not be assigned to home health fieldwork.

Home health usually presents students with a variety of home situations that they have never encountered and may never have imagined. This may include circumstances of extreme poverty, housing conditions that are substandard, including homes with no indoor plumbing, and conditions that are not clean or sanitary. How clients and their families interact with one another, how they treat their possessions, and how they treat their pets may be very different from anything the student has previously encountered. Chapter 5 of this manual describes these aspects of home health in more detail, but it is important that the student be prepared for these aspects of practice and have demonstrated a level of maturity and professionalism to respond to unfamiliar and possibly extreme circumstances.

As mentioned earlier, home health is also a setting that is structured and organized to comply with state and federal regulations and payer criteria. Federal and state requirements regarding criminal background checks, immunizations, and other requirements for health care workers will apply to students who are entering clients' homes or accessing client records. The agency must agree to the fieldwork experience and must establish an agreement with the educational program prior to placement of a student. This may seem obvious, but some occupational therapists in home health function as independent contractors rather than as employees of the home health agency. In other cases, occupational therapy practitioners are employees of a staffing agency that contracts with the home health agency. In these cases, it is not sufficient for the educational program to have a fieldwork agreement with the independent contractor or the staffing company. Federal regulations and voluntary accreditation standards require that the home health agency have oversight of all persons with access to clients or client records. Although independent contractors or staffing agencies may have contracts with the agency, these contracts usually do not include language related to student fieldwork. If an academic fieldwork coordinator wants to establish a fieldwork contract in home health, there should be a formal agreement with the licensed and/or certified home health agency. In cases when an independent contractor or staffing agency is involved, there may also be a second agreement between the educational program and the contractor or staffing agency.

Practitioners and Fieldwork Educators: What You Need to Prepare for Students

For home health practitioners, becoming a fieldwork educator is a respite from the mostly solitary routine of home health practice. Supervising a student is an opportunity to discuss and process care plan expectations and to discuss what is expected and what actually happened during a given home visit. Fieldwork is also an opportunity to recognize, articulate, and reflect on one's tacit knowledge. The presence of a student asking "why" and "how" provides a home health occupational therapy practitioner with an opportunity to talk about the clinical reasoning and decision making that underlie clinical actions. It may be a challenge to mine one's store of knowledge to find answers and to articulate reasons, especially the rationale for actions that are so familiar and common that they feel automatic. Being a fieldwork educator is also an opportunity to be introduced to new knowledge and new ideas drawn from classroom learning shared by the student. For both the practitioner and the student, fieldwork can be a positive experience of learning and professional development.

Being a fieldwork educator involves planning. It is not enough for a student to spend a day, a week, or 12 weeks with you and learn to practice as you do. Fieldwork is not apprenticeship. The goal of fieldwork is to prepare a student to be a generalist entry-level practitioner. This requires planning fieldwork so that the student is exposed to and experiences learning opportunities that prepare him or her for entry-level practice.

Even if you have been a fieldwork educator in another practice setting, fieldwork in home health requires additional planning to account for the decentralized delivery of services. In a facility, students can move from one treatment area to another to observe different clients, different practitioners, and even different disciplines. In home health, these opportunities are not easily accessible, as they occur in different client homes and may be scattered across different neighborhoods and communities. Clients are seen less often than in inpatient settings, and providing a student the opportunity to observe different disciplines working with a single client can be a logistical challenge.

Level I fieldwork experiences require less planning, but it is important to coordinate with the educational program to ensure that the curriculum learning objectives can be met in home health. Level I fieldwork experiences are scheduled in a variety of ways, including intermittent experiences over the course of a semester, regularly scheduled experiences over several weeks, or a full-time weeklong experience. These different fieldwork configurations produce different options for student contact with clients, repeat visits with the same client, and opportunities to observe other disciplines.

If the curriculum objectives are achievable in home health, a Level I experience is an opportunity for you to begin your career as a home health fieldwork educator. A Level I experience requires a more limited commitment of your time and effort, while offering students exposure to home health and offering you the opportunity to acquire and refine your expertise as a fieldwork educator. Level II fieldwork is a much greater commitment of time and effort for a practitioner or fieldwork educator. If you are the only occupational therapy practitioner at your agency, you should consider very carefully the commitment associated with a Level II experience. A Level II experience can be managed by a single practitioner, but it requires a significant commitment prior to the arrival of the student and an intense commitment of your time and effort over the course of the student's experience.

Planning a fieldwork experience begins with expectations and behavioral objectives. If you or your agency has never had a fieldwork student before, then the first step is to formulate these objectives. The simplest way to do this is to start with the fieldwork evaluation. If the proposed fieldwork is Level II, most schools use the standardized fieldwork evaluation, the *Fieldwork Performance Evaluation* (FWPE) (American Occupational Therapy Association [AOTA], 2002a, 2002b). If the proposed fieldwork is Level I, the school should provide its own evaluation tool for the fieldwork site.

The FWPE includes performance criteria in a variety of content areas and domains. These are written generically to apply to a broad range of fieldwork sites. For each of the items on the FWPE, you (and your occupational therapy colleagues at the agency, if any) should develop a corresponding item describing the behavior expected of the fieldwork student. Behavioral objectives should reflect entry-level practice in your home health setting (Wimmer, 2004). In some cases, it may seem that some of the FWPE items do not apply to home health. In these situations, it is best to consider the intent of the FWPE item (e.g., management of equipment and supplies) and write behavioral objectives that meet that intent but are consistent with agency policy and the environment in which such behavior is expected. You should not rule out a FWPE item as "not applicable," as the educational programs determine student grades based on scoring of all the FWPE items. The AOTA has resources for fieldwork on its Web site (www.aota.org), including resources for writing fieldwork objectives and samples of objectives for a variety of sites (though none for a home health setting).

Developing the behavioral objectives is the most time-consuming and thought-provoking aspect of establishing a fieldwork site in home health, but it is not the only task. Once you have established the behavioral objectives, the next step is to develop a schedule for the fieldwork experience. For a Level II experience, the schedule should include orientation to the agency (including any activities or educational activities required for staff members who have contact with clients) and opportunities for the student to interact with other disciplines and to observe services provided by disciplines other than occupational therapy. Particularly in the early weeks of a Level II fieldwork experience, it is less important for the student to spend large amounts of time on visits with you than it is for the student to understand how a home health agency operates and to become familiar with the services provided. If there are other occupational therapy practitioners at your agency, the schedule should include time on visits with those other practitioners so that the student is exposed to the clinical reasoning and practice of more than one practitioner. The schedule should also include any learning activities the student is expected to complete and milestones the student is expected to achieve (e.g., the point at which the student is expected to conduct intervention visits or evaluation visits without the direct participation of the fieldwork supervisor). If your agency has both occupational therapists and occupational therapy assistants, the schedule and milestones should also include the opportunity for an occupational therapy student to be involved in the supervision of an occupational therapy assistant or for an occupational therapy assistant student to collaborate directly with the supervising occupational therapist. The schedule should also include planned time for you and the student to regularly review the student's progress and, if appropriate, to adjust the schedule to optimize learning opportunities for the student.

Whether a student should conduct independent (unaccompanied) home visits is a question that comes up often in reference to home health fieldwork. There is no black-and-white answer to this question that applies uniformly, though in each state the Occupational Therapy Practice Act may include specific requirements for student supervision. In states where there is no such requirement, the prudent response is that students should not conduct independent visits. For detailed information, check your state's Web site. In addition this information can be found on the AOTA Web site (www.aota.org). This recommendation is based on federal home health regulations that define "qualified personnel" and on guidance issued by the Centers for Medicare and Medicaid Services (CMS) and the U.S. Department of Health and Human Services Office of the Inspector General. The federal regulations, known as the

Medicare conditions of participation (CoPs) for home health agencies ("Home Health Services: Personnel Qualifications," 2006), apply to all services provided by Medicare-certified home health agencies, regardless of payer. The CoPs specifically cite definitions for personnel qualified to conduct home health visits; the CoPs do not include students in the list of qualified personnel. The U.S. Department of Health and Human Services Office of the Inspector General (2006) has initiated investigations to verify that home health therapy services provided are necessary and adequately documented and meet all criteria established by Medicare. The number of visits provided by therapy disciplines in a home health episode has an impact on the episode payment, with intense therapy having the effect of nearly doubling the episode payment. Because students are unlicensed personnel who have not yet demonstrated the minimum competencies required to practice occupational therapy, an independent visit made by a student would not meet the requirements for a legitimate therapy visit for episode payment purposes. The AOTA stated, "Services by students can be provided (as allowed by state law) as part of a home health visit, when the student is supervised by an OT or OTA in the home" (AOTA, 2002d).

The CMS (2007) has indicated that it is considering generalizing the student supervision requirement for skilled nursing facilities to all Medicare-regulated settings. In skilled nursing facilities, where Medicare Part A payment also is linked to intensity of therapy services, student services must be provided within "line of sight" supervision of the licensed practitioner.

A licensed practitioner should be present for all visits conducted by a student, with participation of the licensed practitioner gradually reduced over the course of the fieldwork experience as the student demonstrates increasing competence and confidence. Because the presence of the licensed practitioner is more conspicuous in the home setting than in a therapy gym or other facility-based setting, it is reasonable for the licensed practitioner to maintain a "within sight" or "within hearing" presence, even if from an adjacent room, so that the presence of the practitioner does not influence or interfere with the client's response to the student.

There is an additional pragmatic reason for students to be accompanied on all home visits. As previously noted, many home health patients have multiple health conditions. In each year from 2002 to 2005, over 25% of home health patients experienced an acute hospitalization during the home health episode of care (Home Health Quality Improvement Organization Support Center, 2007). Practitioners conducting home visits must be prepared to recognize emergent changes in client status and, if necessary, to communicate with physicians and other disciplines to arrange additional services or to make modifications to the plan of care. Even if a student demonstrated skills that might indicate the ability to conduct an independent visit to implement the established plan of care, expecting a student to identify and respond to emergent changes independently introduces undue risk to both the client and the student.

Home Health Agency Administrators: What You Need to Know to Offer a Fieldwork Experience

Establishing your agency as an occupational therapy fieldwork site offers both short-term and long-term benefits for your agency. In the short term, fieldwork is an opportunity for your agency to develop relationships with occupational therapy educators and educational programs. Fieldwork also expands and strengthens the professional competencies of your occupational therapy staff. In the long term, contributing to the educational experience of occupational therapy students increases the number of occupational therapy practitioners who are aware of home health practice. Establishing relationships with educational programs increases your opportunities to make occupational therapy educators, students, and alumni aware of employment opportunities within your agency. Home health fieldwork expands the supply of entry-level practitioners with both interest and experience in home health.

If your agency already offers clinical education experiences for other disciplines, such as nursing students, you may already have policies and procedures (P&P) in place to ensure that these clinical experiences are in compliance with federal and state home health regulations, accreditation standards, state regulation of the discipline, and educational standards for the discipline. State regulation and educational standards for occupational therapy are not the same as those for nursing, social work, or physical therapy. You should consult your state Occupational Therapy Practice Act and associated rules and regulations to determine whether there are specific requirements related to qualifications of clinical educators or intensity of student supervision. Nationally, occupational therapy educational standards are established by the Accreditation Council for Occupational Therapy Education (ACOTE). Key aspects of the standards for occupational therapy fieldwork education are summarized in Table 6.1.

Your home health agency may contract for occupational therapy services either with a staffing agency or with independent contractors. If this is the case, there must be agreements in place that ensure that all relevant requirements (federal, state, and ACOTE standards) are met and that each party (agency, contractor, and academic institution) is aware of the responsibilities of the other parties. The agreement between your agency and the academic institution should specify the health requirements and background checks that may be required for persons having contact with either patients or patient records. Having the health and background checks specified in the agreement enables the academic institution to inform students of requirements necessary for completion of fieldwork education. All student records, including academic and health records, are protected under the Family Educational Privacy Rights Act and cannot be disclosed by the academic institution without the consent of the student (Family Education Rights and Privacy Act, 2007). Student records disclosed to your agency are confidential and should be maintained with the same level of security as personnel records or patient records.

If your agency does not offer clinical education experiences for other disciplines, then relevant P&P must be developed. Because students are not volunteers, observers, or credentialed practitioners, it is not appropriate to simply apply personnel or volunteer policies to fieldwork students. Because students function in the roles of observer, volunteer, and service provider, it is unlikely that existing P&P for any one of these roles will be appropriate and adequate. Instead of creating a new set of P&P, it is simpler to review existing P&P for both occupational therapy staff and volunteers, identify which of these pertain to students on fieldwork, and revise the wording of those P&P to specifically identify their applicability to students on fieldwork experiences. Occupational therapy practitioners who will serve as fieldwork educators should participate in this process along with personnel familiar with accreditation, certification, and licensure requirements for your agency.

One of the key decisions your agency will make will be whether you will provide Level I fieldwork, Level II fieldwork, or both. Level I demands significantly less preparation and practitioner investment than

TABLE 6.1
Selected Standards and Requirements
for Occupational Therapy Fieldwork Education

Fieldwork experience	Level I	Level II
Purpose	The purpose is to introduce students to the fieldwork experience, to apply knowledge to practice, and to develop an understanding of the needs of clients.	The goal of Level II fieldwork is to develop competent, entry-level, generalist occupational therapists.
Duration	It varies and is commonly scheduled on intermittent dates during a semester or for consecutive days over a shorter span.	The duration is typically 12 weeks (of 24 weeks required).
Intensity	There is no requirement.	It is full-time but may be completed part-time (at least 50% as defined by the agency) for a longer duration equivalent to 12 weeks full-time.
Supervisory credentials	Qualified personnel may include, but are not limited to, currently licensed or credentialed occupational therapists and occupational therapy assistants, psychologists, physician assistants, teachers, social workers, nurses, and physical therapists.	The supervising therapist is a currently licensed or credentialed occupational therapist who has a minimum of 1 year of practice experience subsequent to initial certification and is adequately prepared to serve as a fieldwork educator. The supervising therapist may be engaged by the fieldwork site or by the educational program.
Supervisory intensity	It is not specified.	The supervising therapist ensures that supervision provides protection of consumers and opportunities for appropriate role modeling of occupational therapy practice. Initially, supervision should be direct and then decrease to less direct supervision as is appropriate for the setting, the severity of the client's condition, and the ability of the student.

(Table continues)

(Table 6.1, continued)

Fieldwork experience	Level I	Level II
Relationship between the academic institution the and agency	Responsibilities of the institution and fieldwork site must be clearly documented in a memorandum of understanding. For active Level I and Level II fieldwork sites, programs must have current fieldwork agreements or memoranda of understanding that are signed by both parties. The memorandum of understanding between the institution and the active fieldwork site is reviewed by both parties at least every 5 years.	
Collaboration with the academic program	The academic and fieldwork educators collaborate in establishing fieldwork objectives, identifying site requirements, and communicating about student progress and performance during Level I and Level II fieldwork.	

Note. Based on *Standards and Interpretive Guidelines*, by Accreditation Council for Occupational Therapy Education, 2007, Bethesda, MD, American Occupational Therapy Association. Effective January 1, 2008.

Level II. For this level, the fieldwork objectives and the fieldwork evaluation are developed by the academic program. Schedules for Level I fieldwork vary among educational programs. The most common schedules are (a) regularly through all or part of a semester, for example, every Wednesday for 4 weeks or every Friday afternoon for 3 months and (b) a single full-time week. Half-day experiences may not be compatible with the scheduling and travel aspects of home health, but otherwise Level I is typically a good fit for home health. The goal of Level I fieldwork is "to introduce students to the fieldwork experience, to apply knowledge to practice, and to develop understanding of the needs of clients" (ACOTE, 2006a, p. 12). Students typically have assignments based on their exposure to practice and their contact with patients. These are assigned by the educational program. Common Level I assignments include conducting a patient interview, participating in selected aspects of a patient evaluation or intervention visit under the direct supervision of the occupational therapist, developing a case report or profile, planning and implementing a specific intervention for a patient while directly supervised by a licensed occupational therapy practitioner, observing services provided by other disciplines, and observing a team or case conference. Because supervision by an occupational therapist is not required for Level I, you do not have to have an occupational therapist available full-time to offer a Level I experience.

Level II fieldwork is a significantly greater commitment than Level I in terms of practitioner effort and responsibility. Unlike Level I, Level II is nearly always scheduled as a 12-week full-time experience (based on how "full-time" is defined by the agency) for an occupational therapist student and an 8-week full-time experience for an occupational therapy assistant student. The ACOTE standards permit the completion of an equivalent Level II experience on a part-time basis (at least 50% as defined by your agency policies), but an academic program is unlikely to seek a part-time arrangement unless it is trying to accommodate a student whose specific circumstances require a part-time experience. It is common for educational programs to secure Level II fieldwork bookings many months in advance. Having a site cancel or having to terminate an experience prematurely can adversely affect the scheduled student's ability to graduate in a timely manner. If your agency is contacted about offering a Level II experience, it is important that you have adequate occupational therapy staffing throughout the experience.

Determining Level II fieldwork objectives, student responsibilities, and student assignments is the responsibility of the site (your agency). The objectives should be developed by the occupational therapists serving in the role of fieldwork educator, with input from the educational programs with which your agency has fieldwork agreements. Students are evaluated using the FWPE. The evaluation form is provided to your site by the academic program, but fieldwork objectives should be developed in advance so that the fieldwork educators and the student have a clear understanding of what is expected of the student. Behavioral objectives should be developed by your occupational therapy practitioners to reflect entry-level occupational therapy practice in your setting.

Productivity is a legitimate concern when establishing a home health fieldwork site. Overall there should be little impact on productivity. Because the practitioner and student travel together all day, the time spent traveling provides the "teachable moment" to plan and prepare as well as to process and give and receive feedback. Because the travel time is an existing aspect of home health practice, using this time for student education does not affect practitioner productivity or agency cost. It is advisable that the practitioner and fieldwork educator establish a regular face-to-face meeting schedule (not in the car) to review and plan for the student's learning, but because the car time provides opportunity for immediate feedback, it is unlikely that a regular educator–student meeting should require more than 1 hour per week.

The other aspect of productivity that may arise relates to home visits conducted by a student. Because the CoPs ("Home Health Services: Personnel Qualifications," 2006) do not include students as qualified practitioners, Medicare-certified agencies should not allow or expect students to make unsupervised home visits. For Medicare Part A patients, students may participate in services, and over the course of the fieldwork experience, students should gradually assume responsibility for a caseload as the practitioner's role shifts from leading to coparticipating to monitoring. If your agency provides therapy services under the Medicare Part B outpatient therapy benefit, those visits must be *conducted* by a licensed practitioner. The *Medicare Benefit Policy Manual* stated, "Only the services of the therapist can be billed and paid under Medicare Part B. The services performed by a student are not reimbursed even if provided under 'line of sight' supervision of the therapist; however, the presence of the student 'in the room' does not make the service unbillable" (CMS, 2006, p. 184).

Summary

The goal of fieldwork is to develop competent, entry-level, generalist occupational therapy practitioners. The Institute of Medicine (2003) identified five core competencies for health professionals to meet the needs and demands of 21st-century health care. These five core competencies are to (a) provide patient-centered care, (b) work in interdisciplinary teams, (c) employ evidence-based practice, (d) apply quality improvement, and (e) utilize informatics. All five of these competencies can be addressed in home health fieldwork.

As the demographics of the United States are transformed by the aging of baby boomers and by a growing population with chronic health conditions, home health services will continue to grow. Entry-level practitioners must be prepared to practice in a service delivery system that is shifting away from institution-based inpatient delivery toward decentralized, community-based delivery. Home health fieldwork provides students learning and experience in the home health setting so that they are better prepared to practice in the setting upon completion of their entry-level education. The Medicare home health CoPs permit entry-level occupational therapy practitioners to work for certified home health agencies ("Home Health Services: Personnel Qualifications," 2006), but agencies are more likely to consider an entry-level practitioner who has completed a fieldwork in home health. Informal reports from home health agency administrators indicate that there is a growing gap between the need for occupational therapy practitioners in home health and the supply of such practitioners. Home health fieldwork offers a means to reduce this gap by increasing the number of entry-level practitioners who have experience in the home health setting.

Planning for Discharge

Phyllis L. Ehrlich, MS, OTR/L, CHES

Occupational therapists play a very important part in the process of discharge planning. It is often the occupational therapist who looks ahead to the day when professional service providers will no longer be in the patient's home and the patient must manage safely either independently or with the assistance of a caregiver. He or she is often the professional who can determine how much help the person will require to manage safely within the home. Many times it is also the occupational therapist who initiates a referral for a social worker, as these professionals have many resources to help patients remain at home independently and safely. This chapter will help you plan for discharge from home care and provide ideas on how to make a smooth transition for the patient.

Whether or not you realize it, you begin planning a patient's discharge from the very first visit. Discharge planning must be part of the initial evaluation and should be discussed with the patient and caregiver during the first or second visit. This may seem early, but the reality of home care is that the number of allowable visits is decreasing. At the end of the assessment process, you will use your clinical reasoning skills to assess how much time is needed to achieve the goals you and the patient have set together. Some of this may depend on the complexity of the case and what goals the patient would like to achieve. During the next several weeks, you will be planning ahead to prepare the patient to reenter the community. It is important for patients to recognize that you and other professionals will not be with them forever (as much as some might like this) and that they have only a limited amount of time to achieve their goals. To facilitate this process, practitioners need to be aware of community resources, to build a network of contacts, and to know whom to contact to find out about various options. It is also important to involve the social worker as part of the team to help with this transition and to provide information to the patient.

It is equally important to stay in weekly contact with the other members of the team to find out how the patient is progressing within each discipline. Doing so enables you to coordinate the discharge plans for the patient, whether the person is reentering the community or the person is starting an outpatient therapy program. Remember that once the patient is no longer homebound, then, according to Medicare regulations, home therapy can no longer be provided. (Refer to Chapter 2 for a discussion of Medicare regulations and conditions the patient must meet to qualify for home health care.) Both moral and ethical obligations factor into the decision-making process when treating a patient and planning for discharge. Among these are deciding when a patient has reached maximum potential, providing occupational therapy according to the Occupational Therapy Code of Ethics (American Occupational Therapy Association [AOTA], 2005), and advocating for patients who need continued care in another setting. What this means is that although you may feel that the patient needs further therapy, he or she may no longer be homebound but could benefit from outpatient treatment. This may then involve the social worker to help the patient set up transportation to the outpatient setting.

Discharge Planning

Figure 7.1 contains a checklist that will help you think through the steps of planning discharge, a process that should begin at the first visit.

How do you know when to discharge a patient? As you work to assist your patient toward independence and discharge, remind yourself often just what the goals are for this patient. As each goal is reached, you may want to check it off on your copy of the initial evaluation. This will help you organize your discharge summary and remind you which goals were and were not reached. If you are seeing a patient for a long time, or if you have to give status updates to an insurance company, you may also want to write the date accomplished by each goal on the evaluation.

Planning Aftercare
and Making Appropriate Referrals

It is in patients' best interest for you to prepare them for the reality of life after home care. When you are making recommendations about

Initial Visit

Patient's Name: _____

Record Number: _____

Tasks:	Notes:	Date Completed:
Perform evaluation. Set functional goals with the patient, based on what is important to him or her. Project the number of visits needed to reach those goals. "Plant the seed." Let it be known that you will not be visiting indefinitely (and neither will the home health aide) and that the patient must be prepared for discharge. Recommend additional adaptive equipment or assistive devices to ensure safety in the home during the performance of activities of daily living (ADL) and instrumental activities of daily living (IADL). Plan to involve the caregiver (if there is one) to help the patient reach therapeutic goals.		

Continuing Visits

Tasks:	Notes:	Date Completed:

Figure 7.1. Discharge planning checklist.

aftercare, it is helpful to give the patient and caregivers time to consider them. (Written information may help them in discussing the options and reaching decisions.) Common discharge scenarios include the following:

Outpatient therapy: Outpatient therapy includes occupational therapy services provided in a hospital-based or freestanding clinic to patients who are not homebound.

Home program: This is a written program of exercises or activities that the patient can continue doing independently (see Appendix A for reproducible patient education materials).

Aquatics program: This is a water-based exercise class. Some patients may be able to enroll in a water aerobics class at a local health club (some have senior-adapted classes), and some hospitals or rehabilitation centers offer courses especially for people with disabilities.

Adult day center: This is a structured care setting to which the patient goes during the day (typically 3 to 5 days a week). Adult day centers typically offer activities such as cognitive stimulation, exercise groups, and community outings, and many provide a cooked meal.

Driving evaluation: This is an evaluation to determine whether the patient is a candidate to resume driving and, if so, to provide and teach the patient to use adaptive equipment (e.g., telescope, hand controls). A driving evaluation is often recommended for patients who have had a cerebral vascular accident (CVA), head injury, visual impairment, or cognitive or perceptual deficits. Only a specially trained professional (often an occupational therapist) should perform this evaluation. Look in your telephone directory or contact a local rehabilitation center.

It may be the responsibility of the physician or the insurance company to determine the aftercare plan, and you and the patient may not be involved directly. Still, the recommendations you make in your discharge report will carry weight. In addition, many patients will look to you to explain or direct them to services. (Remember to document and report any recommendations in writing.) Your practice can be enhanced only if you explore and familiarize yourself with the services available in your geographical practice area. (See Appendix B for a list of resources and agencies.)

In Chapter 4 we discussed writing discharge notes organized by goals. Once you have provided this information on the discharge summary, including intervention methods and outcomes, you will want to decide how that patient's progress will affect your aftercare recommendations. If the patient did not reach all of the goals, think about the following questions:

1. What goal or goals were not reached? Why?
2. Can these goals be reached with additional home therapy?
3. Is this patient likely to reach these goals or make progress with outpatient therapy?
4. Is this patient an appropriate candidate for outpatient therapy?
5. Is this patient able to leave the home to travel to outpatient therapy?
6. Is the patient motivated to continue treatment, either at home or as an outpatient? (Sometimes patients are burned out and need a break after receiving therapy in the hospital, in the rehabilitation setting, and then at home.)
7. Does the patient have a support system to assist in achieving his or her goals?

Keeping these questions in mind will help you make decisions about aftercare referrals for the patient. Usually you know the patient well enough by this point to make appropriate aftercare recommendations that will be acted on and followed.

Not every patient will need or is a candidate for outpatient treatment. Sometimes a home program and a caregiver who will help the patient carry it out are sufficient. Whatever the decision is, it should be carefully thought out and discussed with the patient and caregiver.

Providing Patient Education Materials

Patient education materials are of two basic types: (a) background information and resources, and (b) home program activities (see Appendix A for reproducible patient education materials). These written instructions are designed to supplement and reinforce direct instruction in activities that the patient or caregiver can complete without direct therapist supervision (the second category in the hierarchy described in Chapter 5). Tell the patient and caregiver in clear and jargon-free terms what they are to do, including necessary cues or environmental setup. Have both the patient and the caregiver demonstrate the activity so you can ensure that they understand the techniques and are performing the skill correctly. To facilitate their understanding and to allow plenty of time for learning and problem solving, introduce patient education materials as early as possible and review them often.

As discharge approaches, begin providing home program activities designed to help the patient maintain the level of function reached while in home therapy. If any caregivers are frequently present, then also instruct them in the home program so they can encourage and assist the patient to carry it out. Again have the patient and caregiver demonstrate the activities during the session to ensure comprehension.

Providing the home program several weeks or sessions prior to discharge allows time to review it with the patient and ensure that the patient and caregiver are comfortable with it prior to discharge. If the patient progresses during this time, the program can be upgraded. Stress to the patient that it is important to carry through with the home program long term to maintain the current level of function or even make progress after formal treatment ends.

Encourage patients to continue with their home program as long as they feel it is helping them. How long the home program must be continued depends on the nature of the diagnosis. A patient with an acute condition such as a fractured shoulder, for example, would be encouraged to continue the home program until full range of motion has been achieved. In contrast, a patient with a chronic disability following a CVA would be encouraged to perform range-of-motion exercises for his or her lifetime. (Refer to Chapter 4 for a discussion about providing the patient with markers of progress or regression that indicate when occupational therapy reevaluation is appropriate.)

Top 10 Questions Patients and Families Ask

1. How long will it take until I am better?
2. How long will I have to keep doing my home program?

3. Will I be able to drive again?
4. Will I be able to return to my favorite activity [or life role; e.g., going to the senior center, cooking, cleaning the house, etc.]?
5. Why will [the patient] listen to you but not to us? Why does he do the home program for you but not for us?
6. How many times a day do I have to do my exercises?
7. How long will you keep coming here?
8. Can you come back if I get better [or worse]?
9. Should I continue my exercises if they hurt?
10. Does my insurance cover this treatment? How much is this costing me?

During the course of treatment, you may hear one, several, or all of these questions, from either patients or caregivers. Answering them truthfully, to the best of your knowledge, is important. It is best not to take away hope from a patient or loved one but not to provide false hope either.

If I were asked by a man who had had a severe CVA if he would ever use his hand again, I would probably answer this way: "I can't answer that for sure. You won't be able to use your hand like you did before, but you may be able to use it to assist your other hand." If the CVA was relatively recent, I might add, "Your stroke is relatively recent, and you may continue to progress for more than a year and recover the use of your hand." It is important to let patients know that they play important roles in their own recovery. The therapist can instruct and educate them and give them the tools they need to progress, but it is up to them to follow through and to request assistance from a caregiver if it is needed. It is important that patients understand this, as sometimes the patients think that if they do not progress, you will continue to make visits until they are better.

It is also important to involve the caregiver in the discharge process. The caregiver may be responsible for encouraging the patient with the home program, helping the patient perform the activities, or transporting the patient to an outpatient facility. If no caregiver is involved, or the caregiver is unwilling or unable to participate, this must be taken into account when considering aftercare. It is important to identify such cases early in treatment so that appropriate support services can be initiated.

A significant issue in the success of a home program after discharge is consistency. If several caregivers are assisting the patient, then plan to meet with all of them prior to discharge to ensure that they understand the program and correct strategies for assisting the patient with ADL (e.g., the proper method of carrying out a transfer). Perhaps a family meeting can be arranged so that everyone involved in the patient's care can be instructed at once. Teaching one caregiver and expecting that person to pass along the information usually does not work. Trusting caregivers to relay messages can be especially hazardous in the areas of transfers, safety issues, or even range-of-motion exercises, all of which need to be performed in a certain way to protect the patient.

Resolving Ethical Issues in Discharge

During the course of therapy, ethical issues may arise that make the decision to discharge a patient a difficult one. Chapter 4 gives three typical reasons for discharging a patient: goals are met and a functional maintenance program is in place, the patient is no longer homebound, and the patient is rehospitalized for a medical problem. There are, however, at least four other situations that, when properly documented, are legitimate reasons for discharge. These are as follows:

1. The patient is unable to participate in therapy.
2. The patient is not demonstrating progress (what I termed a *nonprogressive patient*).
3. The patient has reached a plateau in treatment.
4. The living arrangement that the patient is in is not safe for the therapist to enter.

Every therapist must set personal limits about when to discharge a patient who does not appear to be benefiting from therapy. Although it is essential to give patients every chance possible to reach their goals, at some point you must know when to stop and discharge them. Continuing to treat a patient who is not making progress may cause the third-party payer to deny coverage for treatment services.

If the patient does not progress or reaches a plateau despite your best therapy, you must document what has occurred during the treatment sessions and explain to the patient and family that you are discharging the patient, along with the reasons why. If the patient is unable to participate in therapy, family members or caregivers can be instructed in a home program. The same is true if a plateau occurs.

If the patient is nonprogressive, however, the decision regarding how long to continue therapy before recommending discharge with a home program may be a difficult one. Another ethical problem often arises in such cases, namely, that the patient and/or family may disagree with your decision to discharge. How can this dilemma be handled? It is important to sit down with the patient and family and explain your decision to discharge, with the reminder that home care can be restarted if there is a significant change in the patient's status—either improvement or decline. You may wish to explain that third-party payers can deny payment for services if progress is not documented.

I encountered a difficulty like this when I received a new referral for an older man I had previously treated for hemiparesis following a CVA. The diagnosis on the second referral was completely unrelated to the CVA. Upon arriving for the initial evaluation, I found that both the patient and the family expected me to continue the previous treatment. I explained that unless the patient's status had declined, treatment could not focus on his arm because he had not had a second CVA. I did in fact find declines in the patient's ADL status and lack of follow-through with the home program. On the basis of these findings, I set up a short-term program to bring the patient back to his prior ADL level and to reinstruct the patient and his family in the home program, while focusing most of the treatment time on the new diagnosis. Once I discussed this plan with the patient and family, they agreed to it.

This leads to the next problem of having to discharge a patient because a third-party payer will not authorize further visits. In my experience this is a rare occurrence, provided you can document the need for services and can speak directly with the case manager. Sometimes it is the physician who refuses to authorize or prescribe therapy. In this case you will want to speak with the physician about his or her reasons for doing so. If you feel strongly that the patient will decline without treatment, explain to the physician exactly how your services can benefit the patient and the probable effect on the patient's functional abilities of receiving versus not receiving occupational therapy. Emphasize how your services are valuable to the patient and will improve the person's quality of life.

Whenever treatment is denied, the therapist and family need to advocate for the patient by any means possible, including contacting the physician, the insurance company, the case manager, and whoever else might have input. Unfortunately most home health agencies instruct therapists not to continue treating patients without approved visits. If you continue to treat the patient while the case is appealed, you risk not being reimbursed for your services if the case is denied. Be prepared to submit documentation or appear before the insurance review board to fight your case.

You will rarely encounter a patient who is not living in a safe situation. This may mean that it is not safe for the therapists or other members of the team to visit the patient. This can range from something as simple as a flea infestation in the house (which obviously needs to be treated) or something as serious as an abusive person living with or visiting the patient. There was a case like this that involved a patient who had been living in her own house and had a son who visited often. Unfortunately he was abusing drugs and was occasionally violent with his mother, although she would not admit this. After her hospitalization, she went to stay with her daughter for several weeks but then decided she wanted to return home. The social worker was involved and tried to persuade her to stay with her daughter, but the patient was very insistent about returning home. Because she would not admit that her son had hit her, we could not initiate a referral for adult protective services, and we had to let her return home. However, we decided that services would not continue once she returned home because we felt it was an unsafe situation to place any members of the team into.

Improving Follow-Through

When discharge is imminent and the home program has been provided to the patient and family, what can you do if you have concerns that the family may not follow through with the maintenance program? Part of your strategy will be to try to prevent this problem. During the course of treatment, you have established a rapport with the patient and the family. You have brought the patient to a higher level of functioning, building a relationship of trust. Because you provided the patient and family with the home program several weeks ahead of time, you can continually check in with them to monitor how well the program is being carried out. If follow-through is poor, you may want to try to arrange a session with a family member who can be responsible for carrying out the home program with the patient. If this is not feasible, attempt to adjust the program so the patient can carry it out independently. Emphasize how important it is to carry out the home program if the patient wishes to maintain the quality-of-life gains attained through therapy. It may be reassuring to remind the patient and family that home therapy can be restarted if there is a significant change in the patient's status. There are no guarantees that a home program provided will be carried out. As the therapist, you hope that you have created a strong enough rapport with the patient and family that they will recognize it is clearly in the patient's best interest to follow through with maintenance.

Even with the patient's best intentions, it takes discipline to follow through with a home program once the structure of regular therapy has ended, particularly if the patient has recovered sufficiently to resume a number of life activities. It is helpful to work with the patient to identify ways to integrate maintenance exercises into the daily routine so they become a habit. For example, can some exercises be done during the commercial breaks in the patient's favorite television programs? Can the patient do a few range-of-motion stretches while reaching to dust picture frames or put away dishes? Recruiting friends and relatives to offer reminders and encouragement may help patients who tend to be depressed or forgetful.

Addressing Safety Concerns

Another concern prior to discharge is ensuring that safety issues have all been adequately addressed. Safety concerns need to be addressed almost from the first visit. It is important to involve the family and caregiver in this instance, presenting them with the risks and the solutions to the problems. Patients and families do have a choice about heeding your recommendations. After listening to your concerns and suggestions, they still may choose not to make the recommended changes. In these cases, you must document the discussion, your concerns and recommendations, and the outcomes or choices of the patient and family. This will cover you legally if any problem should arise. It also is wise to leave a written copy of safety recommendations with the patient in case he or she chooses to make changes later on, after discharge. Place a copy of your recommendations in the patient's chart with your documentation.

Occasionally you will have to perform an accelerated discharge: a safety check that is completed within one or two sessions. Because a safety check involves only one or two visits, discharge planning must start from the initial phone call. You need to immediately start building rapport with patients so they will be more amenable to your recommendations. A few minutes of conversation on the phone when setting up the initial visit will give you an idea of the patient's abilities, lifestyle, and important activities.

Once at the house, you will want to have the patient accompany you from room to room, discussing what functional activities take place there and where difficulties arise. You may want to have the patient demonstrate transfers into and out of the tub or shower and on and off the toilet or bed, obtain needed objects from cabinets, and use the microwave or stove. Perhaps spend one session in the kitchen having the patient prepare a hot beverage and transport it to the table or wherever he or she might drink it and having the patient prepare a simple snack or lunch. As you move through the home, you can make safety suggestions, taking into account that the patient has probably lived there a long time and is used to things being a certain way. Like anyone else, patients may have idiosyncratic ways of doing certain things, and as long as their way is safe, it may be what works best for them.

It is very important to leave your recommendations in writing, perhaps listing your safety concerns as well. Place a copy in the patient's agency chart.

Leave your name and the phone number of the agency in case the patient wants to reach you to ask further questions. Also leave information on how to contact durable medical equipment dealers. In the case of an accelerated discharge, you may not have an opportunity to find out whether the patient makes changes or purchases equipment. On the other hand, you may be surprised when a patient phones you weeks or even months later to tell you about an equipment purchase. The patient may wish instruction in the use of that equipment, which can be arranged with a physician's order.

Community Resources

As part of helping patients prepare for discharge into the community, be it in a short time or after several weeks of home therapy, you should be aware of other resources and information that we can provide them. Becoming familiar with community resources includes such issues as knowing where patients can go for outpatient therapy or an aquatics program, how to put them in contact with social service agencies, and where they can find support groups appropriate to their disability. Other important issues include the following:

- What does the patient need to do to apply for handicapped license plates? Typically one must contact the American Automobile Association (AAA) or the state's Department of Motor Vehicles. Many programs that offer driving evaluations and intervention also have the necessary paperwork. The patient's physician typically must provide medical information and verify the application.
- How can the patient apply for public transportation for people with disabilities? This may involve a free or reduced-cost bus pass or transportation in a wheelchair-equipped van, depending on the services available in your area and the patient's needs.
- How does the patient contact the Meals on Wheels program? Depending on your area, this service may be run by a private charity, such as a church group, or by a government-sponsored agency. It is important to stay apprised of the current cost for this service and know whether a sliding fee scale is available, as cost may be an issue for patients on a fixed income.

These issues are usually the professional responsibility of a social worker, but sometimes you are placed in the position of dealing with them. Getting a referral to social work authorized is sometimes difficult, so it is helpful if you can provide general information to the patient or the family. A general knowledge of available social services may also help in justifying a referral to social work. You may also find that patients ask you questions they do not ask anyone else because of their rapport with you. Not every patient will request this type of information, but for the ones who do, it is useful to have information on hand or know where to find it. Sometimes this is as simple as pulling out the telephone directory to help a patient solve the problem of where to find products or services. This activity can be incorporated into a treatment session, especially with patients who have cognitive deficits, to help them learn to use a telephone directory and find community resources. If you offer such information to a patient or caregiver, document the specifics and leave a copy in the home for the information of other team members and caregivers.

Case Examples

Two case studies are presented to illustrate the process of discharge planning.

Case 1: Helen

Helen, an 80-year-old woman, fell at her son's home and fractured her left shoulder. She received a hemiarthroplasty of the left shoulder. At the time of referral for home occupational therapy, she was allowed to move her left arm but required moderate assistance for her ADL and IADL. She was unable to transfer to the shower independently or do any of the cooking, both of which she valued and wished to resume.

The occupational therapy treatment plan included instruction in shower transfers, self-care activities, and kitchen activities. Performance skill-based intervention included range-of-motion exercises and activities to help her regain more functional use of her left arm. She was provided with a detailed home program to perform on nontherapy days. Her progress in this area was slow, and I notified the physician of progress with notes sent with the patient on two of her medical appointments.

By the end of 6 weeks of home therapy, she was no longer homebound, had progressed to being independent in shower transfers and self-care activities, and had resumed some of her occupational roles, such as cooking and doing the dishes. Her use of her left arm was not progressing as quickly as the physician or I would have liked, however. I recommended a referral to outpatient occupational therapy, and both the physician and Helen concurred. I provided the names of several outpatient facilities. I also recommended a maintenance program to help Helen maintain her independence in self-care and provided her with written markers she could use to identify loss of function or increased safety risks in this area. Helen was encouraged to bring any concerns to her physician and the occupational therapist who would take over her outpatient therapy.

Case 2: Carol

Carol, a 66-year-old woman, had rheumatoid arthritis, hypertension, coronary artery disease, syncope (blackouts), and Cushing's disease. Upon discharge from the hospital, she was referred for home care. Upon making a home visit with the physical therapist, we found Carol on the floor, with facial lacerations, contusions, and ecchymosis (bruising). We phoned an ambulance, fearing the worst (hip fracture, stroke, or both). She was admitted to the hospital with a diagnosis of syncope. Upon her release, new physical and occupational therapy consultations were ordered.

Carol's goals were to return to the level of independence in ADL and IADL she had experienced prior to this latest hospitalization. Carol actively participated in designing her intervention plan, with an understanding that occupational therapy visits were limited. Increasing Carol's occupational performance through environmental changes and therapeutic activities facilitated a successful discharge. We started by ordering bathroom equipment that would enable her to shower independently. She purchased a transfer bench, a handheld shower, and a grab bar, the latter two being installed by the vendor. I then instructed Carol in transfers so she could safely get into and out of the shower by herself.

The next challenge to tackle was the kitchen. After assessing the kitchen, I requested that the maintenance service at her apartment complex switch the handles on her refrigerator to the other side. This would make it easier for Carol to open the refrigerator and transfer items she was removing or replacing to adjacent counter space.

From here, we moved on to cooking some simple meals and preparing and transporting a hot beverage. I made several suggestions to help Carol be more independent in the kitchen and more safely transport her meals out to the living room, where she liked to eat. An insulated travel mug allowed her to transport a hot beverage without spilling it. She also obtained a walker basket. This enabled her to place her hot meals in a plastic sealable container, which she then placed in the walker basket to transport. She also learned to use a long-handled reacher to obtain needed objects from cabinets and the refrigerator.

The final area of concern for Carol was being able to do her laundry in the laundry room, which was directly across from her apartment. Although she was unable to transport a laundry basket, she was able to gather a load of clothes in a plastic bag, which she balanced on top of her walker basket along with her detergent. After starting the washing machine, she returned to her apartment to rest until the wash cycle was finished. She then returned to place the wash in the dryer, using her long-handled reacher to retrieve clothing from both the washer and the dryer. I instructed Carol in energy-conservation and work-simplification techniques to prevent her from getting short of breath or fatigued during this activity, and I provided patient education materials. Although Carol did not require any other adaptive devices, I provided information and phone numbers for local arthritis organizations in the event that she wanted support or further information about her rheumatoid arthritis. I provided Carol with written markers to help her identify problems or loss of function. With these, Carol could notify her physician and request further occupational therapy if her condition deteriorated.

The final component of the discharge plan was Carol's decision to purchase a Lifeline emergency response system because she was afraid of falling or having another syncopal episode. She was discharged from occupational therapy, having met her goals of returning to her previous level of independence in ADL and IADL.

Conclusion

As you can see, it is important to begin thinking about the discharge from day one of the initial evaluation. Your planning for the patient's aftercare may depend on many factors: physicians, insurance companies, families, the patients themselves, and other contributing circumstances. Your suggestions are important, and your clinical expertise is invaluable when making recommendations. If you listen to your patients in normal conversation, you will undoubtedly hear what is important in their lives. You can use that knowledge to help them plan and achieve many of their goals prior to discharge.

After you spend several sessions with a patient, you will want to see him or her continue to progress without you. Therefore take everything into account before you make suggestions. Make sure what you recommend is in the best interest of the patient. Offering several options is usually the best plan and empowers the patient to make informed decisions. Patients do have a say in their aftercare and, whether or not you agree with their ideas, it is critical that they be considered when decisions are made unless you feel it may jeopardize their safety. In that case it is best that you explain how and why their decision may endanger them.

When the day of discharge comes, we can know that we have done our best if we have helped the patient prepare for a productive and safe future.

Appendix A
Patient Education Materials

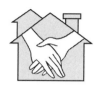

Catherine Verrier Piersol, MS, OTR/L
and Phyllis L. Ehrlich, MS, OTR/L, CHES

The following patient education materials (represented in this appendix as thumbnails) are contained on the accompanying CD-ROM:

Shoulder and Elbow Exercises and Activities
Forearm, Wrist, and Hand Exercises and Activities
Arthritis Exercises
Putty Exercises
Resistive Band Exercises
Reducing Hand Swelling
Improving Hand Dexterity
Moving Your Arm on Your Own
Increasing Environmental Awareness
Getting Dressed Below the Waist:
    Pants and Socks
Getting Dressed Above the Waist:
    Button-Down Shirt, Method 1
Getting Dressed Above the Waist:
    Button-Down Shirt, Method 2
Getting Dressed Above the Waist:
    Pullover Shirt
Positioning Yourself in Bed After a Stroke
Performing Daily Activities After Your Hip Replacement
Taking Care of Your Joints
Making Daily Activities at Home Easier
Ideas for One-Handed Home Management
Going Out Into the Community
The Americans With Disabilities Act (ADA)
Ensuring Your Safety at Home

This appendix contains thumbnails of the reproducible patient education materials provided on the CD-ROM. The forms are prepared handouts that are designed to increase efficiency, but the following features still allow for individualization:

- At the beginning of each form is an identification area with space for the patient's name and medical record number, your agency's name and phone number, and your name and phone number.
- There are boxes for checking off items the patient should read or do.
- There is a section at the end of each form titled "Just for You" that provides the therapist plenty of space to write comments and individualized procedures and activities.

The patient education materials are occupation based and consist of *home programs* and *information sheets*. The home program materials are divided into two categories: performance skills (motor and process skills) and occupational performance areas (self-care and home management). The information sheets focus on context issues (community travel and safety). All home programs and information sheets are provided on the CD. We used large print to accommodate patients with low vision. For ease of organization, consider printing the pages on different colors of paper to designate the type of information, for example, home programs that focus on performance components versus ones that target occupational performance areas.

Occupational Therapy Home Program

Name _____ Record # _____
Agency _____ Phone # _____
Therapist's Name _____ Phone # _____

Shoulder and Elbow Exercises and Activities

These exercises will help increase the movement and strength of your arms so you can perform your daily activities better.

Please do the exercises checked (✓) below. Do each exercise _____ times. Repeat _____ times a day.

You can do these exercises while either sitting or standing.

Precautions
1. Do not hold your breath while doing these exercises.
2. Stop immediately if you feel discomfort or pain; notify your therapist or physician or both.

Shoulder Exercises

Therapist's Comments:

☐ Shrug your shoulder upward, downward, and in a circle.

☐ Sit or stand facing a wall. Place your open palm on the wall in front of you. "Walk" your fingers up the wall as far as you can. Try to reach a little higher each day.

☐ Lace your fingers behind your head so that your elbows are bent out to the side. Bring your elbows together in front of your face as close as you can, then take them back out to the side. (Do not strain your neck.)

☐ Begin with your arms at your sides. Raise your arms out to the side and as high over your head as you can. Try to touch your palms together over your head. (This movement looks like making a "snow angel.")

Shoulder and Elbow Exercises and Activities

Occupational Therapy Home Program

Name _____ Record # _____
Agency _____ Phone # _____
Therapist's Name _____ Phone # _____

Forearm, Wrist, and Hand Exercises and Activities

The following exercises and activities will increase the movement and strength of your forearms, wrists, and hands so you can perform your daily activities better.

Please do the exercises checked (✓) below. Do each exercise _____ times. Repeat _____ times a day.

You can do these exercises while either sitting or standing.

Precautions
1. Do not hold your breath while doing these exercises.
2. Stop immediately if you feel discomfort or pain. Notify your therapist or physician or both.

Forearm and Wrist Exercises

Therapist's Comments:

☐ Rest your hand sideways on the table, with the little finger resting on the table. Bend your wrist forward and backward.

☐ Rest your forearm on the table with your hand hanging over the edge. Slowly raise and lower your hand. (To improve your strength, hold a small can while you do this.)

☐ Hang your hand over the edge of the table, turning it sideways so your little finger is toward the floor. Move your hand up and down as if shaking hands or hammering a nail. Keep your forearm resting on the table so the movement is at your wrist.

Forearm, Wrist, and Hand Exercises and Activities

Occupational Therapy Home Program

Name _____ Record # _____
Agency _____ Phone # _____
Therapist's Name _____ Phone # _____

Arthritis Exercises

These exercises will increase your arm function so you can do your daily activities better.

Please do the exercises checked (✓) below. Do each exercise _____ times. Repeat _____ times a day.

Do these exercises sitting at a table in a supportive chair.

Precautions
1. Do these exercises only when you are feeling up to it.
2. Do not do these exercises if your joints are inflamed (swollen).
3. Do not hold your breath while doing these exercises.
4. Stop immediately if you feel discomfort or pain. Notify your therapist or physician or both. These exercises can be modified for you.

Arthritis Exercises

Therapist's Comments:

☐ Place a towel on the table in front of you. Place both hands on the towel. Slide the towel away from you and bring it back using your open hands. Do this _____ times. Repeat the set _____ times.

☐ Place a towel on the table in front of you. Place both hands on the towel. Slide the towel to the left, then to the right _____ times using your open hands. Repeat the set _____ times.

☐ Place a towel on the table in front of you. Place both hands on the towel. Slide the towel in a clockwise circle _____ times. Change direction and repeat _____ times. Repeat the set _____ times.

Arthritis Exercises

Occupational Therapy Home Program

Name _____ Record # _____
Agency _____ Phone # _____
Therapist's Name _____ Phone # _____

Putty Exercises

These exercises will increase the strength in your hands so you can perform your daily activities better.

Please do the exercises checked (✓) below. Do each exercise _____ times. Repeat _____ times a day.

Precautions
1. Do not hold your breath while doing these exercises.
2. Stop immediately if you feel discomfort or pain. Notify your therapist or physician or both.

Putty Exercises

Therapist's Comments:

☐ Squeeze the putty in your _____ hand.

☐ Roll the putty out into a log shape. Pinch the putty between your _____ thumb and each finger, one at a time.

Putty Exercises

Occupational Therapy Home Program

Name _____ Record # _____
Agency _____ Phone # _____
Therapist's Name _____ Phone # _____

Resistive Band Exercises

These exercises will increase your strength and endurance so you can perform your daily activities better.
    Please do the exercises checked (✓) below. Do each exercise _____ times. Repeat _____ times a day.

Precautions
1. Do not hold your breath while doing these exercises.
2. Stop immediately if you feel discomfort or pain. Notify your therapist or physician or both.

Band Exercises

Therapist's Comments:

☐ While sitting in a chair, hold the ends of the band in your hands and pull straight across your chest. You will look as if you are pulling taffy.

☐ Place one hand in your lap in front of your hip and hold the band. Hold the other end of the band with the opposite hand and pull upward at a diagonal. You will look as if you are pulling a sword out of a sheath. Switch sides.

Resistive Band Exercises

Occupational Therapy Home Program

Name _____ Record # _____
Agency _____ Phone # _____
Therapist's Name _____ Phone # _____

Reducing Hand Swelling

It is difficult to do everyday activities with a swollen hand. Your hand may hurt and your fingers cannot easily grasp and work with objects. The following methods will reduce the swelling in your hand and allow pain-free movement.

Precautions
1. Follow the procedures exactly to ensure positive results.
2. Stop immediately if you feel discomfort or pain. Notify your therapist or physician or both.
3. Please use only the method(s) that your occupational therapist has showed you and checked (✓) below.

Methods

Therapist's Comments:

☐ Do an ice bath _____ times per day.
1. Fill a basin with ice water (3/4 ice, 1/4 water).
2. Submerge your _____ hand in the ice water.
3. Hold your hand in the water for 5 seconds. Remove your hand for 15 seconds.
4. Repeat this process for no more than 10 minutes.

☐ Use an ice pack or bag of frozen vegetables (peas, corn) _____ times per day.
1. Place your _____ palm down on the table.
2. Gently place the ice pack or bag of frozen vegetables directly on the back of your hand. Leave it there for no more than 10 minutes.

Reducing Hand Swelling

Occupational Therapy Home Program

Name _____ Record # _____
Agency _____ Phone # _____
Therapist's Name _____ Phone # _____

Improving Hand Dexterity

You probably have trouble handling small objects because your fingers are weak or move slowly. This makes it difficult to do everyday activities, such as buttoning your shirt, brushing your teeth, or opening a pill bottle. The following activities will improve your hand coordination to make daily tasks easier to do.
    Perform the activities checked (✓) below _____ times a day.

Precautions
1. Do not hold your breath while doing the exercises.
2. Stop immediately if you feel discomfort or pain. Notify your therapist or physician or both.

Hand Dexterity Exercises

Therapist's Comments:

☐ Pick up coins of various sizes and turn them over from head to tail and back again. After turning them over, pick them up and place them in a container without sliding them to the edge of the table.

☐ Pick up toothpicks with your fingers without sliding them to the edge. Now try picking them up with tweezers!

☐ Practice picking up playing cards off a table without sliding them to the edge.

☐ Pinch clothespins and clip them on the edge of a can or plastic container or on a yardstick. Then remove them.

☐ Tap one finger at a time against a table. Begin with your index finger and move to your little finger, then reverse direction.

Improving Hand Dexterity

Occupational Therapy Home Program

Name _____ Record # _____
Agency _____ Phone # _____
Therapist's Name _____ Phone # _____

Moving Your Arm on Your Own

The following exercises and activities will maintain movement, prevent stiffness and swelling, and increase awareness of your _____ arm and hand.
    Please do the exercises checked (✓) below. Do each exercise _____ times. Repeat _____ times a day.

Precautions
1. Breathe evenly while doing the exercises.
2. Stop immediately if you feel discomfort or pain. Notify your therapist or physician or both.
3. Do these exercises slowly.

Shoulder Exercises

Therapist's Comments:

☐ Clasp your hands or cradle your arms together. Reach forward with your arms and lift them above your head as high as you can.

☐ Clasp your hands or cradle your arms together. Raise your arms to shoulder height and move them from side to side.

Moving Your Arm on Your Own

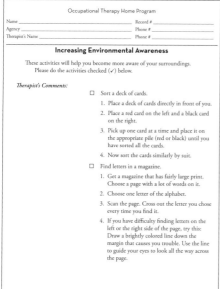

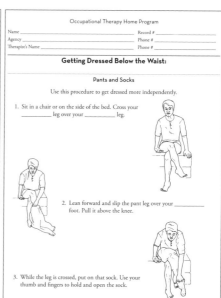

Increasing Environmental Awareness

Getting Dressed Below the Waist:
Pants and Socks

Getting Dressed Above the Waist:
Button-Down Shirt, Method 1

Getting Dressed Above the Waist:
Button-Down Shirt, Method 2

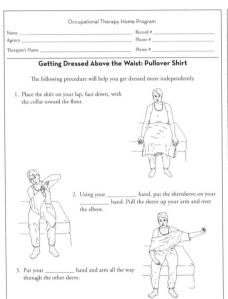

Occupational Therapy Home Program

Name _____ Record # _____
Agency _____ Phone # _____
Therapist's Name _____ Phone # _____

Getting Dressed Above the Waist: Pullover Shirt

The following procedure will help you get dressed more independently.

1. Place the shirt on your lap, face down, with the collar toward the floor.

2. Using your _____ hand, put the shirtsleeve on your _____ hand. Pull the sleeve up your arm and over the elbow.

3. Put your _____ hand and arm all the way through the other sleeve.

Occupational Therapy Home Program

Name _____ Record # _____
Agency _____ Phone # _____
Therapist's Name _____ Phone # _____

Positioning Yourself in Bed After a Stroke

After your stroke you may find you have weakness or difficulty moving that keeps you from lying comfortably in bed. These tips will help you position yourself in bed. Several positions are suggested so you can find one or two positions that are comfortable and enable you to fall asleep. You may need help positioning some of the pillows to get them in the right places.

Lying on Your Back

Place one pillow under your shoulders. Place a rolled towel or pillow under your pelvis. The pillow under your shoulder may be the same one you use for your head. Place another pillow next to your body on your weaker side. Extend your arm out to the side on the pillow.

Lying on Your Weaker Side (the _____ side)

Lie on your side, making sure your weaker shoulder blade is in contact with the bed. Place a pillow in front of your belly and put your stronger arm on it. You may place another pillow between your legs. Slide your top hip forward and rest your knee and ankle on that pillow.

Getting Dressed Above the Waist: Pullover Shirt

Positioning Yourself in Bed After a Stroke

Occupational Therapy Home Program

Name _____ Record # _____
Agency _____ Phone # _____
Therapist's Name _____ Phone # _____

Performing Daily Activities After Your Hip Replacement

After a hip replacement, you must follow certain important precautions. You will not be able to move your new hip in certain ways for a period of time. Because of these precautions, you may have to do daily activities a little differently than you used to. Here are some guidelines to follow.

Note. Always do exactly what your surgeon tells you, even if it is a little different from these instructions.

☐ You have received the following adaptive equipment:

  ☐ Reacher
  ☐ Dressing stick
  ☐ Long-handled shoehorn
  ☐ Sock donner
  ☐ Long-handled sponge
  ☐ Other _____

Please follow the suggestions checked (✓) below.

☐ When getting dressed, sit on a sturdy surface (bed or chair). Use your adaptive equipment to help you put on your underwear, pants, socks or stockings, and shoes.

☐ When taking a shower (not a bath), it is safest to sit on some type of chair. Use a long-handled sponge to wash your lower legs and feet. Ask your occupational therapist where you can purchase a shower chair.

Occupational Therapy Home Program

Name _____ Record # _____
Agency _____ Phone # _____
Therapist's Name _____ Phone # _____

Taking Care of Your Joints

It is important to keep your joints active but in a way that will not cause further damage. These are called joint-conservation (saving) techniques. Using these techniques means you will have to do things differently than you are used to, and they may take some extra time. This is not always easy to do. But if you stick with it, your efforts will pay off in the long run.

Why Do I Need to Care for My Joints?

• If you have arthritis, it is very important to make a conscious effort to protect your joints.

• Protecting your joints prevents unnecessary strain and damage.

• These techniques may lessen your pain and will help you retain the use of your arms and hands.

How Do I Get Started?

• Many of these suggestions are common sense, and you may already be doing them.

• Some of the suggestions are new and unfamiliar. It may take you a little while to get used to them.

• Don't be afraid to experiment with ways to protect your joints. Use these ideas as guidelines but adapt them to fit your lifestyle.

• If something does not work the first time, try it again. If it still does not work, try another method.

• Don't be afraid to ask for help from family, friends, or neighbors.

• If you keep trying, you will succeed. And your joints will thank you for it!

Performing Daily Activities After Your Hip Replacement

Taking Care of Your Joints

Occupational Therapy Home Program

Name _____ Record # _____

Agency _____ Phone # _____

Therapist's Name _____ Phone # _____

Making Daily Activities at Home Easier

By simplifying tasks and saving your energy, you can get more done and feel better.

What Are Work Simplification and Energy Conservation?

Work simplification means breaking down tasks to their simplest form to avoid unnecessary steps.

Energy conservation helps you save your strength. You can use shortcuts, good body mechanics, and appropriate planning techniques to do things more efficiently.

How Do I Get Started?

Use these ideas and think of others to help you conserve your energy and simplify your work in many different areas.

☐ Conserving your energy will allow you to do other things that are really important to you.

☐ Always plan ahead with everything you do and take your time. You will find you can get more done in ways that do not make you as tired.

☐ Remember to take frequent rest breaks, breathe properly, and don't overdo it.

☐ You will find you have more energy and enjoy life a little bit more!

Making Daily Activities at Home Easier

Occupational Therapy Home Program

Name _____ Record # _____

Agency _____ Phone # _____

Therapist's Name _____ Phone # _____

Ideas for One-Handed Home Management

As you become able to resume some of your household activities, follow these ideas, which will make doing these activities as easy as possible.

How Do I Get Started?

• Before beginning any task, plan ahead.

• Think about what supplies you will need to complete the task and gather them before you start.

• Have someone nearby if you think you may need help.

• When doing something you haven't tried for a while, it may be helpful to talk through what you will do (step-by-step) before actually doing it.

How Do I Use These Ideas in My Daily Life?

Please refer to the items checked (✓) below. These suggestions will help you perform activities in an easier way.

Kitchen

☐ Use a wheeled utility cart to gather everything you need for meal preparation. This will not only save steps but keep everything you need together. Use the cart when setting the table, preparing a meal, and cleaning up.

☐ When buying a utility cart, make sure it will roll easily on all kinds of surfaces (carpets and bare floors).

☐ Look for appliances you can use with one hand, such as the following: electric knife, electric can opener, wire whip, flour sifter, jar opener, egg separator, one-handed egg beater, and rolling pin.

Ideas for One-Handed Home Management

Occupational Therapy Information Sheet

Name _____ Record # _____

Agency _____ Phone # _____

Therapist's Name _____ Phone # _____

Going Out Into the Community

Once you are finished with your home care visits, you may want to go out and have some fun! Here are a few ways to make it easier and safer to leave your home.

How Will I Get Where I Want to Go?

• Take advantage of handicapped parking spaces. You can apply for a special license plate through your state Department of Motor Vehicles.

• Your doctor must complete a form that verifies you are able to drive and need handicapped parking.

• Consider using public transportation. Many cities provide van transportation for people with disabilities.

• Use a taxi if you can afford it.

• Ask a friend or relative to drive in exchange for your buying a meal or doing something in return.

What Should I Find Out Before I Go Someplace?

Phone ahead and confirm that you can access the places you want to visit. Here are some questions to ask:

• Are there steps?

• If so, how many?

• Are there ramps or an elevator?

• Is there assistance for people with disabilities?

• Where is the parking lot located?

• Is handicapped parking or valet parking provided?

Going Out Into the Community

Occupational Therapy Information Sheet

Name _____ Record # _____

Agency _____ Phone # _____

Therapist's Name _____ Phone # _____

The Americans With Disabilities Act (ADA)

You have certain rights under the ADA. The areas covered include employment (getting and performing a job), public accommodations (getting to and entering public places), transportation (accessing and using public transportation), telecommunications (using telephones and communication devices), and state and local governments (accessing and using governmental offices and information).

Employment

• As of July 26, 1992, employers with 15 or more employees had to comply with the ADA requirements.

• An employer cannot discriminate against you in hiring or promotion because of your disability if you are qualified for the job.

• During a hiring interview, the employer may ask about your ability to perform a specific task required on the job but may not ask if you have a disability.

• Employers may not ask you to perform tests or tasks that would screen out someone with a disability.

• Employers are required to provide "reasonable accommodations" to enable you to perform your job. This may include modifying equipment or structuring the job differently. Employers may be exempted if they can show this imposes an "undue hardship" on the operation of the business.

Public Accommodations

• As of January 26, 1992, restaurants, retail stores, and hotels cannot discriminate against people with disabilities.

• Accommodations must be provided to anyone with hearing or vision impairment or other disability, unless it would result in an undue burden.

• All new construction and facilities must be accessible.

• Physical barriers in existing facilities must be removed or an alternative method of providing services must be offered.

The Americans With Disabilities Act (ADA)

Occupational Therapy Information Sheet

Name _____ Record # _____

Agency _____ Phone # _____

Therapist's Name _____ Phone # _____

Ensuring Your Safety at Home

Maintaining a hazard-free home environment helps you get around your home and do your daily activities. Consider the ideas checked (✓) below.

General Suggestions

☐ Have emergency phone numbers next to all the telephones in your home.

☐ If you have a programmable phone, put emergency numbers in memory.

☐ Get rid of unnecessary throw rugs in your home. Use nonskid backing on throw rugs that are absolutely necessary.

☐ If you have a fireplace, have a barrier (screen or doors) in place.

☐ Avoid multiple electrical connections or multiple extension cords.

☐ Install light switches at both the bedroom door and your bedside (or put a touch plate on your bedside lamp).

☐ Use nightlights in hallways, bedrooms, and bathrooms.

☐ Keep all bureau drawers and cabinet doors closed so you don't bump into them.

☐ Mark sliding glass doors with decals so they are easy to see.

☐ Keep passageways clear.

☐ When climbing stairs, use a handrail at all times.

☐ You may want handrails on both sides of the stairs for more safety.

Ensuring Your Safety at Home

Appendix B
Resources

It is important to be aware of and utilize resources that are available to you and your patients. The following resources offer pertinent information and can answer some of the questions you and your patients may have regarding home health care.

Contact Information

Administration on Aging
www.aoa.dhhs.gov
American Association for Homecare
www.aahomecare.org
American Association of Nurse Assessment Coordinators
www.aanac.org
American Hospital Association
www.aha.org
American Medical Association
www.ama-assn.org
American Occupational Therapy Association
www.aota.org
American Physical Therapy Association
www.apta.org
American Public Health Association
www.apha.org
American Speech-Language-Hearing Association
www.asha.org
Case Management Society of America
www.cmsa.org
Centers for Medicare and Medicaid Services
www.cms.hhs.gov

Centers for Medicare and Medicaid Services Home Health
Agency Center
www.cms.hhs.gov/center/hha.asp

Family Caregiver Alliance
www.caregiver.org

Health Industry Distributors Association
www.hida.org

Health Information Portability and Accountably Act
www.cms.hhs.gov/HIPAAGenInfo

Joint Commission on Accreditation of Healthcare
Organizations (JCAHO)
www.jcaho.org

National Association for Home Care and Hospice
www.nahc.org

National Family Caregivers Association
www.nfcacares.org

National League for Nursing
www.nln.org

Outcome and Assessment Information Set (OASIS)
www.cms.hhs.gov/OASIS/

U.S. Department of Health and Human Services
www.os.dhhs.gov

U.S. Department of Justice
www.usdoj.gov

Agencies and Services

Other services vary from state to state or community to community.
The following is a list of the general types of agencies and services that
are widely available and may assist your patients.

Adult Day Centers: These centers may be run by private
agencies, hospitals, or city governments. They provide supervised activities and often hot meals during the day.

Adult Protective Services/Older Adult Protective Services:
This is the agency to contact if you have confirmed that

a patient is experiencing any kind of abuse, neglect, or exploitation. Some states operate a toll-free hotline.

Agency on Aging: This state- or city-run organization may have a waiting list. It can provide a whole host of services from day care programs, homemakers, and home health aides to therapy or equipment.

Associated Services for the Blind: This organization offers talking books, talking clocks, magnifiers, and many other devices to help individuals with visual problems.

Foundations and Societies: These organizations (e.g., the Arthritis Foundation) often assist qualified individuals with the cost of durable medical equipment, assistive devices, and home modifications.

Geriatric Psychiatric Services: Psychiatric help or counseling is available for individuals older than age 60 years who have mental health problems.

Meals on Wheels: This organization delivers hot meals to homebound people for a small fee. Either food will be delivered daily or a week's worth of meals will be delivered in reheatable containers. Usually milk, fruit, juice, and sandwich fixings are provided in addition to the hot meal.

Transportation Services: Special public transportation services can be set up for people unable to use the regular bus service by applying through the local public transportation system. There is often a small fee for use.

Local Resources

There are many state associations of medical equipment suppliers. You may want to search the Web for your state association of medical equipment suppliers.

Glossary

Abuse: Abuse is the willful physical and/or psychological mistreatment of a patient, usually by a caretaker. It includes verbal or emotional mistreatment of a patient.

Activities of daily living (ADL): ADL are basic activities of daily living that consist of self-care tasks; for example, bathing, dressing, grooming, and eating.

Aftercare: Aftercare is the period of time directly following the termination of home care services during which some form of follow-up service is provided. Aftercare may consist of medical, therapeutic (outpatient), or community-based services.

Areas of occupation: Areas of occupation is the division of daily occupations into activities of daily living, play and leisure activities, and work or productive activities.

Balanced Budget Act of 1997 (Public Law 105-33): This legislation was signed into law by President Bill Clinton in August 1997. The intent of the BBA is to balance the federal budget and maintain solvency of the Medicare program.

Care path: A care path is a protocol that anticipates a patient's course of treatment, based on diagnosis and/or problem area, prior to admission to the home care agency. It is also referred to as a clinical pathway, team plan, diagnostic treatment plan, or comprehensive plan of care.

Caregiver: In the context of this manual, the caregiver is the individual involved in providing assistance, care, and support to the patient on a daily basis (typically a relative or friend with no professional training in therapy).

Centers for Medicare and Medicaid Services (CMS): The CMS is the federal agency that administers Medicare, Medicaid, and child health insurance programs. The majority of recipients receive their benefits through the fee-for-service delivery system, but an increasing number are choosing managed care plans.

Client factors: These are the underlying factors that contribute to one's ability to complete daily occupations, including sensorimotor components (sensory, neuromusculoskeletal, motor), cognitive components, and psychosocial skills and psychological abilities.

Community Health Accreditation Program (CHAP): This is a not-for-profit organization that evaluates and accredits home health agencies. CHAP has a cooperative accreditation agreement with the Joint Commission on Accreditation of Healthcare Organizations (JCAHO). The accreditation policies and procedures for CHAP are comparable to and accepted by JCAHO.

Conditional reasoning: Conditional reasoning is a form of clinical reasoning in which the practitioner considers the patient's unique circumstances and conditions and uses this information to help the patient envision his or her future.

Contexts: Contexts are the situational factors that influence occupational performance, comprising temporal aspects (chronological, developmental, life cycle, and disability status) and environmental aspects (physical, social, cultural).

Diagnosis-related group (DRG): A DRG is a classification of illnesses and injuries used to determine payment for hospital-based treatment.

Durable medical equipment (DME): DME is equipment and supplies that are deemed medically necessary, including wheelchairs, walkers, canes, commodes, and oxygen.

Environmental contexts: Environmental contexts are the physical, social, and cultural contexts that influence occupational performance.

Evidence-based practice: This is the process of assessing and utilizing current research information to design and implement intervention.

Exploitation: A caregiver's use of his or her influence over a patient for personal gain, typically resulting in neglect of the patient's needs, is exploitation.

Fiscal intermediary: A fiscal intermediary is a public or private agency or organization that establishes an agreement with the Health Care Financing Administration to process and monitor Part A and Part B Medicare claims for participating providers.

Generalization: Generalization is one's ability to apply learned concepts and behaviors to new and unfamiliar situations.

Health Insurance for the Aged and Disabled Act: This legislation is Title XVIII of the Social Security Act of 1935, signed into law by President Lyndon Johnson in 1965. This legislation established Medicare as the federally funded and administered health insurance program for most individuals age 65 and older.

Homebound: A patient's being homebound is a criterion for receiving home care services based on Medicare guidelines. The service recipient must be confined to the home; the patient need not be bedridden, but leaving the home must require extreme effort (leaving the home for doctor's appointments is permitted).

Informed consent: Informed consent is consent given by a prospective service recipient to receive services after that individual has been provided with information outlining the benefits and the risks of the care to be provided.

Instrumental activities of daily living (IADL): IADL are activities other than basic activities of daily living (ADL) that relate to the ability to manage independently at home; for example, doing laundry, shopping, and managing money.

Interactive reasoning: Interactive reasoning is a form of clinical reasoning in which the practitioner interacts directly with the patient through interview and conversation to better understand the personal experiences of the patient. These insights are used to design patient-centered intervention and identify the patient's goals and significant activities.

Joint Commission on Accreditation of Healthcare Organizations (JCAHO): The JCAHO is an independent, not-for-profit organization that evaluates and accredits more than 19,500 health care organizations in the United States. Its mission is to improve the safety and quality of health care provided to the public, using the practice standards established by each professional organization.

Level I fieldwork: Level I fieldwork includes practicum experiences that occupational therapy students complete while involved in the didactic (classroom) portion of the curriculum. The experience is typically observational in nature with supervised participation.

Level II fieldwork: Level II fieldwork is a full-time (or equivalent) practicum experience that occupational therapy students must complete to meet the requirements to graduate and sit for the National

Board for Certification in Occupational Therapy (NBCOT) certification exam. The student is expected to have skills to serve as an entry-level occupational therapy practitioner by the completion of the fieldwork experience.

Level of assistance: This is a 6-point scale outlined in Medicare guidelines used to describe the patient's level of ability in performing functional transfers and activities of daily living. The levels are total assistance (unable to perform any part of the task), maximum assistance (performs 25% of the task), moderate assistance (performs 50% of the task), minimal assistance (performs 75% of the task), standby assistance (performs 100% of task with supervision for safety), and independent status (performs 100% of task).

Medicaid: Medicaid is a program jointly funded by the U.S. federal and state governments that provides medical insurance to low-income and needy people. Recipients include children or people who are aged, blind, or disabled.

Medicare: Medicare is a program funded by the U.S. federal government that provides health care coverage for people age 65 and older and those with certain disabilities. It is divided into two related health care programs: hospital insurance (Part A) and supplementary medical insurance (Part B). Part A covers inpatient hospital care, home health care, and care in a skilled nursing facility. Part B covers hospital outpatient programs, doctor's fees, home health, and comprehensive outpatient rehabilitation facilities (CORF) fees. It also covers other professional fees.

Neglect: Neglect is the mistreatment through the withholding of basic necessities such as care, food, or medicine.

Nonprogressive patient: A nonprogressive patient is a patient whose progress is limited by physical, psychological, or familial problems such that therapy must be discontinued.

Occupational performance: Occupational performance is the performing of daily occupations.

Occupational profile: An occupational profile is a client-centered approach to understanding what is important and meaningful to the patient and to identifying past experiences and interests that may assist problem solving and guide interventions.

Outcome and Assessment Information Set (OASIS): The OASIS is a questionnaire used to measure patient outcomes in home health for the purpose of outcome-based quality improvement.

Prior level of functioning: Prior level of functioning is the qualitative description of the patient's functional abilities immediately prior to the onset of the current illness or disability.

Procedural reasoning: Procedural reasoning is a form of clinical reasoning in which the occupational therapy practitioner utilizes specific assessment and intervention procedures to determine the disability status of the patient.

Prospective payment system (PPS): The PPS is a system for predetermining the Medicare payments to home health agencies mandated in the Balanced Budget Act of 1997. When implemented, it will provide home health agencies a payment for each 60-day episode of care for each beneficiary. It is adjusted for the health condition and care needs of each beneficiary and for the geographical differences in wages for home health agencies across the country.

Self-management: Self-management is the individual's ability to manage the symptoms, treatment, physical and psychosocial consequences, and lifestyle changes inherent in living with a chronic condition. "Efficacious self-management encompasses ability to monitor one's condition and to effect the cognitive, behavioral, and emotional responses necessary to maintain a satisfactory quality of life" (Barlow, as cited by Glasgow, Davis, Funnell, & Beck, 2003, p. 563).

Self-management support: Self-management support is the process of making and refining multilevel changes in health care systems (and the community) to facilitate [patient self-management] (Barlow, as cited by Glasgow et al., 2003, p. 563).

Third-party payer: A third-party payer is the entity that reimburses the service provider for medical and health services rendered to an individual, when the individual does not pay for services directly (e.g., Medicare, Medicaid, health insurance company, or managed care organization).

References

Abreu, B. C. (2002). Getting started in evidence-based practice. *OT Practice, 7*(18), CE-1–CE-8.

Acceptance of patients, plan of care, and medical supervision. (2002). Conditions of participation for home health agencies. *42 Code of Federal Regulations* 484.18.

Accreditation Council for Occupational Therapy Education. (2006a). *Accreditation standards for a master's-degree-level educational program for the occupational therapist.* Bethesda, MD: American Occupational Therapy Association.

Accreditation Council for Occupational Therapy Education. (2006b). *Accreditation standards for an educational program for the occupational therapy assistant.* Bethesda, MD: American Occupational Therapy Association.

Accreditation Council for Occupational Therapy Education. (2007). *Standards and interpretive guidelines.* Bethesda, MD: American Occupational Therapy Association.

American Medical Association. (2008). *International classification of diseases, 9th revision, clinical modification.* Chicago: Author.

American Occupational Therapy Association. (2002a). *Fieldwork Performance Evaluation for the Occupational Therapy Assistant Student.* Bethesda, MD: Author.

American Occupational Therapy Association. (2002b). *Fieldwork Performance Evaluation for the Occupational Therapy Student.* Bethesda, MD: Author.

American Occupational Therapy Association. (2002c). *Occupational Therapy Practice Framework*: Domain and process. *American Journal of Occupational Therapy, 56,* 609–639.

American Occupational Therapy Association. (2002d). *OT/OTA student supervision and Medicare requirements.* Retrieved October 12, 2007, from http://www.aota. org/Educate/EdRes/Fieldwork/StuSuprvsn/38386.aspx

American Occupational Therapy Association. (2005). Occupational therapy code of ethics. *American Journal of Occupational Therapy, 59,* 639–642.

American Occupational Therapy Association. (2008). *Evidence-based practice resources directory.* Retrieved March 17, 2008, from http://www.aota.org/Educate/ Research/Evidence.aspx

Americans With Disabilities Act of 1990, 42 U.S.C. § 12101 *et seq.* (1990).

Balanced Budget Act of 1997, H.R. 2015, 105th Cong. (1997) (enacted).

Cahaba Government Benefit Administrators. (2006). *Coverage guidelines for home health agencies* [Brochure]. Des Moines, IA: Author.

Centers for Medicare and Medicaid Services. (1999, January 25). *Federal Register, 64*(15), 3764.

Centers for Medicare and Medicaid Services. (2002). *Outcome-based quality improvement (OBQI) implementation manual.* Washington, DC: U.S. Government Printing Office.

Centers for Medicare and Medicaid Services. (2003). *Medicare benefit policy manual.* Retrieved from http://www.cms.hhs.gov/Manuals/IOM/list.asp

Centers for Medicare and Medicaid Services. (2006). Practice of physical therapy, occupational therapy, and speech-language pathology: Therapy students (Publication 100-2, Chapter 15, Section 230). *Medicare benefit policy manual.* Baltimore, MD: Author.

Centers for Medicare and Medicaid Services. (2007). Medicare Program; Revisions to payment policies under the physician fee schedule, and other Part B payment policies for CY 2008; Revisions to the payment policies of ambulance services under the ambulance fee schedule for CY 2008; and the Amendment of the e-prescribing exemption for computer generated facsimile transmissions; Final rule. *Federal Register, 72*(227), 66222–66578.

Clark, F. A. (1993). Occupation embedded in real life: Interweaving occupational science and occupational therapy. *American Journal of Occupational Therapy, 47,* 1067–1078.

Community Occupational Therapists and Associates Health. (2006). *SAFER-HOME* (Vol. 3). Toronto: Author.

Family Educational Rights and Privacy Act. 20 U.S.C. § 1232g. Family Educational Rights and Privacy; Under what conditions is prior consent required to disclose information? (2007). *32 Code of Federal Regulations* 99.20.

Feys, H., De Weerdt, W., Verbeke, G., Steck, G. C., Capiau, C., Kiekens, C., Dejaeger, E., Van Hoydonck, G., Vermeersch, G., & Cras, P. (2004). Early and repetitive stimulation of the arm can substantially improve the long-term outcome after stroke: A 5-year follow-up study of a randomized trial. *Stroke, 35*(4), 924–929.

Glasgow, R. E., Davis, C. L., Funnell, M. M., & Beck, A. (2003). Implementing practical interventions to support chronic illness self-management. *Joint Commission Journal on Quality and Safety, 29*(11), 563–574.

Health Care Financing Administration. (1998). *Medicare outpatient physical therapy and comprehensive outpatient rehabilitation manual* (HCFA Pub. 9). Washington, DC: U.S. Government Printing Office.

Holm, M. (2000). Our mandate for the new millennium: Evidence-based practice; 2000 Eleanor Clarke Slagle lecture. *American Journal of Occupational Therapy, 54,* 575–585.

Holm, M. B. (2001). AOTA continuing education article: Our mandate for the new millennium; Evidence-based practice. *OT Practice, 6*(12), CE-1–CE-16.

Home Health Quality Improvement Organization Support Center. (2007). *Public quality measure data.* Retrieved January 3, 2008, from http://www.hhqi-star.org/star_index.aspx?controls=publicData

Home health services: Personnel qualifications. (2006). *42 Code of Federal Regulations* 484.4.

Institute of Medicine. (2001). *Crossing the quality chasm: A new health system for the 21st century.* Washington, DC: National Academy Press.

Institute of Medicine. (2003). *Health professions education: A bridge to quality.* Washington, DC: National Academy Press.

Jongbloed, L., Stacey, S., & Brighton, C. (1989). Stroke rehabilitation: Sensorimotor integrative treatment versus functional treatment. *American Journal of Occupational Therapy, 43,* 391–397.

Kielhofner, G. (2005). Research concepts in clinical scholarship—scholarship and practice: Bridging the divide. *American Journal of Occupational Therapy, 59,* 231–239.

Law, M. (2000). Evidence-based practice: What can it mean for me? *OT Practice, 5,* 16–18.

Law, M., Baptiste, S., Carswell, A., McColl, M. A., Polatajko, H., & Pollock, N. (1994). *Canadian Occupational Performance Measure* (2nd ed.). Toronto: Canadian Association of Occupational Therapists.

Law, M., Cooper, B. A., Strong, S., Stewart, D., Rigsby, P., & Letts, L. (1996). The *Person–Environment–Occupation Model:* A transactive approach to occupational performance. *Canadian Journal of Occupational Therapy, 63,* 9–23.

Law, M., & MacDermid, J. (2008). *Evidence-based rehabilitation: A guide to practice.* Thorofare, NJ: Slack.

Law, M., Polatajko, H., Baptiste, W., & Townsend, E. (1997). Core concepts of occupational therapy. In E. Townsend (Ed.), *Enabling occupation: An occupational therapy prespective.* Ottawa: Canadian Association of Occupational Therapists.

Lieberman, D., & Scheer, J. (2002). AOTA's evidence-based literature review project: An overview. *American Journal of Occupational Therapy, 56,* 344–349.

Nelson, D. L., Konosky, K., Fleharty, K., Webb, R., Newer, K., Hazboun, V. P., Fontane, C., & Licht, B. C. (1996). The effects of an occupationally embedded exercise on bilateral assisted supination in persons with hemiplegia. *American Journal of Occupational Therapy, 64,* 639–645.

Piersol, C. V. (2005, March). Integrating evidence-based practice in home health. *Home and Community Health Special Interest Section Quarterly, 12,* 2–4.

Quality Insights of Pennsylvania. (2007). *Best practice intervention package: Patient self-management.* Retrieved January 8, 2007, from http://www.homehealthquality.org/hh/hha/interventionpackages/patient_sm.aspx

Ranke, B. A. E. (1998). Documentation in the age of litigation. *OT Practice, 3,* 2024.

Richardson, W. S., Wilson, M. C., Nishikawa, J., & Hayward, R. S. (1995). The well-built clinical question: A key to evidence-based decisions. *ACP Journal Club, Evidence-Based Medicine for Better Patient Care, 123,* A-12.

Robertson, S. C. (1998). Why we document. In *Effective documentation for occupational therapy* (2nd ed.). Bethesda, MD: American Occupational Therapy Association.

Rosenberg, W., & Donald, A. (1995). Evidence-based medicine: An approach to clinical problem-solving. *British Medical Journal, 310,* 1122–1126.

Sackett, D. L., Richardson, W. S., Rosenburg, W., & Haynes, R. B. (1997). *Evidence-based medicine: How to practice and teach EBM.* New York: Churchill Livingstone.

Sackett, J. K., Strauss, S. E., Richardson, W. S., Rosenberg, W., & Haynes, R. B. (2000). *Evidence-based medicine: How to practice and teach EBM* (2nd ed.). Edinburgh, Scotland: Churchill-Livingstone.

Schkade, J. K., & Schultz, S. (1992). Occupational adaptation: Toward a holistic approach for contemporary practice, Part 1. *American Journal of Occupational Therapy, 46,* 829–837.

Schultz, S., & Schkade, J. K. (1992). Occupational adaptation: Toward a holistic approach for contemporary practice, Part 2. *American Journal of Occupational Therapy* [AOTA], *46,* 917–925.

Shaughnessy, P. W., Crisler, K. S., Schlenker, R. E., & Hittle, D. F. (1998). *Outcomes and Assessment Information Set (OASIS B-1).* Denver, CO: Center for Health Services and Policy Research.

Siebert, C. A. (1997a). A description of fieldwork in the home care setting. *American Journal of Occupational Therapy, 51*(6), 423–429.

Siebert, C. A. (1997b). Understanding who "they" are: Regulations governing home health care practice. *Home and Community Health Special Interest Section Quarterly* [AOTA], *4*(4), 2.

Social Security Act, Title XVIII Health Insurance for the Aged and Disabled Act of 1965, U.S.C. §§ 1395-1395ccc, subchapter XVIII, chapter 7, Title 42.

Stube, J. E., & Jedlicka, J. S. (2007). The acquisition and integration of evidence-based practice concepts by occupational therapy students. *American Journal of Occupational Therapy, 61,* 53–61.

Tickle-Degnen, L. (1999). Organizing, evaluating, and using evidence in occupational therapy practice. *American Journal of Occupational Therapy, 53,* 537–539.

Tickle-Degnen, L. (2000a). Communicating with clients, family members, and colleagues about research evidence. *American Journal of Occupational Therapy, 54,* 341–343.

Tickle-Degnen, L. (2000b). Gathering current research evidence to enhance clinical reasoning. *American Journal of Occupational Therapy, 54,* 102–105.

Tickle-Degnen, L. (2000c). Monitoring and documenting evidence during assessment and intervention. *American Journal of Occupational Therapy, 54,* 434–435.

Tickle-Degnen, L. (2000d). What is the best evidence to use in practice? *American Journal of Occupational Therapy, 54,* 218–221.

U.S. Department of Health and Human Services Office of the Inspector General. (2006). *Review of billing under the home health prospective payment system for therapy services* (A-07-04-01010). Retrieved October 2, 2007, from http://oig.hhs.gov/oas/reports/region7/70401010.htm

Vance, K., & Siebert, C. (2007). New competencies in home health. *OT Practice, 12*(13), CE-1–CE-8.

Walker, C. M., Sunderland, A., Sharma, J., & Walker, M. F. (2004). The impact of cognitive impairment on upper body dressing difficulties after stroke: A video analysis of patterns of recovery. *Journal of Neurology, Neurosurgery, and Psychiatry, 75*(1), 43–48.

Walker, M. F., Drummond, A. E. R., & Lincoln, N. B. (1996). Evaluation of dressing practice for stroke patients after discharge from hospital: A crossover design. *Clinical Rehabilitation, 10,* 23–31.

Wallenbert, I., & Jonsson, H. (2005). Waiting to get better: A dilemma regarding habits in daily occupations after stroke. *American Journal of Occupational Therapy, 59,* 218–224.

Wimmer, R. (2004). *Writing site-specific objectives for the FWPE forms.* Retrieved October 10, 2007, from www.aota.org/Educate/EdRes/Fieldwork/SiteOBj/38271

World Health Organization. (2001). *International classification of functioning, disability and health.* Geneva, Switzerland: Author.

About the Authors

Catherine Verrier Piersol (editor) received her bachelor of science degree in occupational therapy from Tufts University, Boston School of Occupational Therapy, and her master of science degree in occupational therapy from Boston University. She is currently enrolled at Virginia Commonwealth University pursuing her PhD in health-related science. Cathy most recently assumed the position of clinical director of the Living Laboratory for Elder Care at the Jefferson Center for Applied Research in Aging and Health (CARAH) at Thomas Jefferson University, after many years as director of the Occupational Therapy Program at Philadelphia University. Throughout her career she has consistently worked in direct service, and she spent the past 10 years working in home care and the community. Cathy served on the Home and Community Health Special Interest Section of the American Occupational Therapy Association from 2004 to 2006. She is active in her local and state associations and regularly presents at local, state, and national conferences.

Phyllis L. Ehrlich (editor) earned her bachelor of science degree in occupational therapy from Temple University and her master of science degree in health education from Arcadia University in Glenside, Pennsylvania. She is NDT trained and is a certified health education specialist. She currently works for Holy Redeemer Home Care in Philadelphia. Phyllis has a regular column in *ADVANCE for Occupational Therapy Practitioners* called "House Calls" and was also published in Home Health Care Management and Practice. She has presented at numerous state, national, and international conferences on a variety of topics. With over 21 years of home care experience, she is also seeing clients to recommend home modifications for safety and accessibility.

Carol Siebert (contributor) received her master of science degree in occupational therapy from the University of North Carolina at Chapel Hill. A home care occupational therapist for 19 years, she has presented on home care issues at state, regional, national, and international occupational therapy conferences. She currently provides in-home occupational therapy services in a community health program for low-income seniors. She is also adjunct assistant professor in the Division of Occupational Science at the University of North Carolina at Chapel Hill. She was a chairperson of the American Occupational Therapy Association Home and Community Health Special Interest Section (HCHSIS) and an editor of the *HCHSIS Quarterly*. She is a fellow of the American Occupational Therapy Association and the recipient of the North Carolina Occupational Therapy Association Suzanne C. Scullin Award, the association's highest award for outstanding practice and contributions to the profession. Carol is currently the president of the North Carolina Occupational Therapy Association.

Karen Vance (contributor) is an occupational therapist with home care experience as a provider, clinical, and regulatory manager since 1981. Karen currently provides clinical and general operations consulting services to home care agencies with BKD Health Care Group. She has presented home care seminars for numerous national, regional, and state associations and several national media organizations for over 15 years. Karen served on the Technical Expert Panel for CMS's Home Health Quality Improvement Campaign in 2007, has contributed to several publications on home care for the American Occupational Therapy Association, and has served as chair of the Home and Community Health Special Interest Section. Karen earned her bachelor of science degree in occupational therapy in 1978 from the University of Missouri, Columbia.